Easy Home Exercises For Seniors Over 60

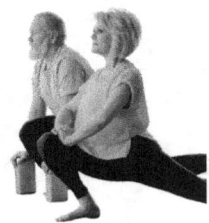

Chair Yoga with Strength Training to Lose Weight and Gain Flexibility

Brian L. Lopez

All rights reserved. No part of this publication may be reproduced, distributed, or transmitted in any form or by any means, including photocopying, recording, or other electronic or mechanical methods, without the prior written permission of the publisher, except in the case of brief quotations embodied in critical reviews and certain other noncommercial uses permitted by copyright law.

Copyright © Brian L. Lopez 2024

TABLE OF CONTENTS

Why This Book?..5
The Benefits of Staying Active After 60...9
A Holistic Approach: Weight Loss, Strength, and Flexibility.....................................13
Chair Yoga and Strength Training: A Perfect Combination......................................17
Chapter 1: The Power of Gentle Movement..23
How Exercise Enhances Longevity and Well-being..23
Common Exercise Myths for Seniors..26
The Impact of Chair Yoga on Flexibility and Pain Relief..29
Strength Training for Everyday Functionality...33
Chapter 2: Getting Started Safely and Smartly...37
Consulting Your Doctor: Exercise Readiness..37
Understanding Your Body's Needs: Flexibility vs. Strength....................................40
Setting Realistic Fitness Goals: Weight Loss and Beyond.....................................43
Creating a Comfortable Space at Home for Exercise and What You'll Need.........48
Chapter 3: Chair Yoga for Beginners..51
What is Chair Yoga?...51
Breathing and Mindfulness Techniques..54
Simple Chair Yoga Poses for Flexibility..59
Seated Cat-Cow Stretch...63
Seated Forward Bend...65
Gentle Chair Twist..68
Seated Mountain Pose..72
Chair Yoga Flow: A 10-Minute Routine to Start Your Day......................................75
Chapter 4: Strength Training with Chairs and Light Weights.................................79
Why Strength Training is Vital After 60..79
How to Use Weights Safely..81
Seated Leg Lifts...89
Chair-Assisted Squats..92
Bicep Curls with Light Weights...94
Overhead Press from the Chair..98
Seated Side Leg Raises...101
Creating a Simple Strength Routine for Muscle Maintenance..............................104
Chapter 5: Stretching for Flexibility and Pain Relief...108
Importance of Stretching for Seniors..108
The Best Stretches for Mobility and Joint Health...111
Neck Stretch...115
Shoulder and Arm Stretch..118
Lower Back Stretch..121
Hip Flexor Stretch...125

- **Seated Hamstring Stretch**...127
- **Building a Stretching Routine for Flexibility and Pain Prevention**.................130
- **Chapter 6: A Balanced Diet to Support Weight Loss and Fitness Goals**........135
- **Nutrition Basics for Seniors: Supporting an Active Lifestyle**..........................135
- **How Diet Impacts Weight Loss and Energy Levels**..138
- **Creating Simple, Healthy Meals**..141
- **Recipes for Weight Loss and Energy**...144
- **Low-Carb Meals**..144
- **High-Protein Snacks**..148
- **Anti-Inflammatory Smoothies**...151
- **Chapter 7: Putting It All Together: A 4-Week Exercise Plan**...........................156
- **Week 1: Getting Acquainted with Movement**...156
- **Week 2: Increasing Strength and Flexibility**..160
- **Week 3: Building Endurance and Weight Loss**..166
- **Week 4: Maintaining Your Progress**..170
- **How to Track Your Success: Weight, Flexibility, and Strength Gains**............174
- **How to Make Exercise a Daily Habit**...178
- **Staying Connected: Encouraging Friends or Family to Join You**...................181
- **Conclusion**..185
- **Bonus**..186
- **Free Workout Videos**...186
- **INDEX**..187

Why This Book?

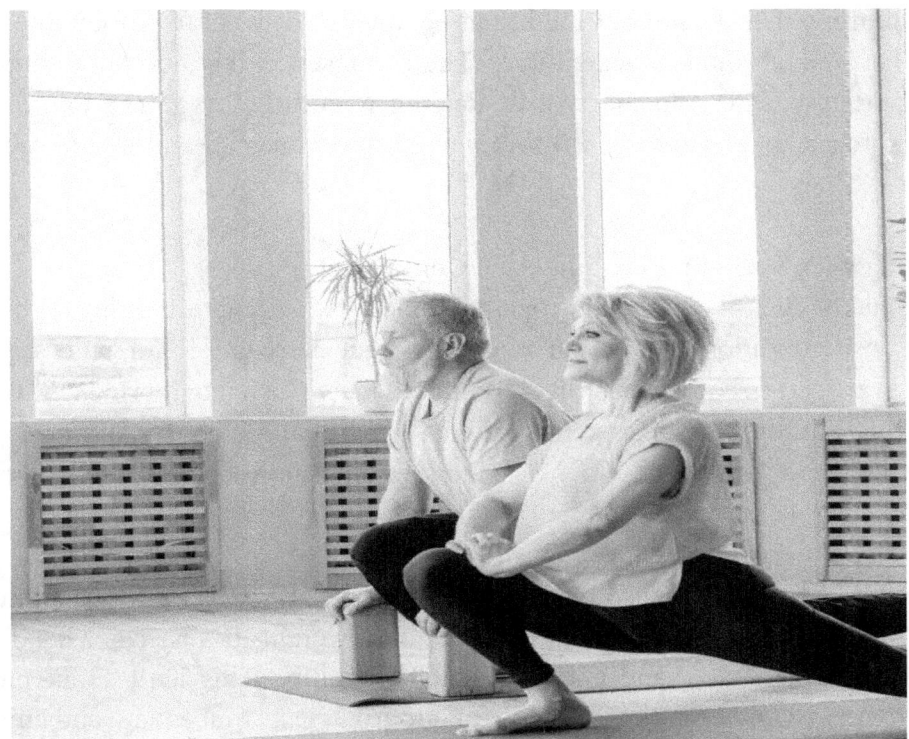

As a fitness instructor with decades of experience helping people of all ages, I've witnessed firsthand the transformative power of movement. But as I worked with more seniors, I realized something important: the mainstream fitness world often overlooks the unique needs of older adults, particularly those over 60. Exercise routines and diets designed for younger bodies can feel overwhelming or, worse, potentially harmful for seniors. Many times, I've met individuals who want to stay active, lose weight, and improve their flexibility but don't know where to start. This book exists because staying healthy, strong, and flexible after 60 is not only possible—it's essential. And it doesn't require intense workouts, high-impact routines, or complicated equipment.

Let me tell you why this book is different and why it was created specifically for YOU.

The Challenge: Exercise and Aging
As we age, our bodies go through natural changes: muscles may weaken, joints stiffen, balance may become a bit trickier, and for many, weight management becomes more challenging than it used to be. It's not that our bodies can't handle exercise, but the way we exercise needs to be adjusted. A 20-year-old can jump into a vigorous HIIT workout or head to the gym for heavy weightlifting. But for someone over 60, who may be dealing with joint pain, arthritis, or even years of inactivity, those same activities can feel more daunting than empowering.

This is where this book comes in. It was designed to address the very specific needs of seniors who want to improve their health but might not be able to (or want to) follow the fitness trends that are popular among younger generations. The exercises in this book are simple, effective, and, most importantly, safe. Whether you're dealing with mobility issues, joint discomfort, or just haven't exercised in a while, you'll find that these routines are tailored to meet you where you are.

The Goal: Aging with Strength, Flexibility, and Confidence
The central focus of this book is chair yoga combined with strength training. Why chair yoga? Because yoga in its traditional form can sometimes feel inaccessible to seniors, particularly if you've never practiced it before or struggle with balance. Chair yoga brings all the benefits of yoga—flexibility, mindfulness, relaxation—into a format that feels safer and more manageable. You don't have to get down on the floor or contort yourself into complicated positions. All you need is a sturdy chair, some space, and the willingness to move.

And why strength training? Because muscle mass declines naturally as we age, but that doesn't mean it's lost forever. Strength training, even with light weights or resistance bands, can reverse muscle loss, improve balance, and enhance overall mobility. This isn't about building bulky muscles; it's about staying strong enough to lift your groceries, climb stairs, and enjoy your daily life with less effort and more confidence.

This book is about more than just exercise routines—it's about building the strength and flexibility that allows you to live independently and confidently. It's about equipping you with the tools to manage your weight, ease joint pain, improve your balance, and regain the energy you once had. Through these exercises, you will gain flexibility in both your body and your mind, learning to move with ease and grace even as the years pass.

Tailored for Real Life: A Sustainable, Flexible Plan
One of the main reasons why seniors struggle to stick with traditional exercise programs is that they often feel overwhelming or unsustainable. That's another reason why I wrote this book. I wanted to create a resource that you can actually stick to, a program that feels like it's enhancing your life, not taking over it. The routines outlined here can be done at home, with minimal equipment, and can easily fit into your daily schedule. Whether you have 10 minutes in the morning or 30 minutes in the afternoon, you can find a routine in this book that meets your needs.

The structure is simple: you'll start with basic chair yoga stretches and gradually incorporate strength training using light weights or resistance bands. There are no long or intense workouts to dread—just short, effective routines that improve your body's functionality, help you lose weight, and boost your flexibility. These exercises are designed for real life. You won't be left feeling sore, exhausted, or frustrated. Instead, you'll feel empowered, energized, and ready for the next day.

Weight Loss Without the Pressure
Let's be honest: weight loss over 60 isn't the same as it was when we were younger. But that doesn't mean it's impossible. This book approaches weight loss in a sustainable, stress-free way. By focusing on building muscle and increasing flexibility, you'll naturally improve your metabolism, burn calories, and shed extra pounds. And because these routines are low-impact, you won't feel like you're punishing your body in the process. Instead, you'll build a foundation of strength and endurance that will make daily activities feel easier, while supporting long-term weight loss.

Additionally, I've included dietary tips that align with the needs of seniors. I'm not talking about restrictive, one-size-fits-all diets. The nutrition guidance in this book emphasizes balance, helping you fuel your body with the right nutrients for energy, muscle recovery, and weight management—all without feeling deprived.

Designed by Experience, Built for Results
I wrote this book after years of working with seniors in fitness classes and one-on-one settings. I've seen the struggles many face: fear of injury, frustration with slow progress, or simply not knowing where to start. I also know the joy and pride that comes when someone realizes they can move more easily, feel stronger, and even lose weight—at any age.

This book is a distillation of everything I've learned from those experiences. It's crafted with care, empathy, and expertise, designed to give you real, lasting results. I'm not just handing you a list of exercises and wishing you luck. I'm guiding you through a program that's been proven to work for seniors just like you.

What This Book Can Do for You
In this book, you'll find a comprehensive program that's more than just a series of exercises. You'll learn how to:

Improve your flexibility and range of motion using simple chair yoga poses designed for seniors.
Strengthen your muscles with easy-to-follow strength training exercises that require minimal equipment.
Lose weight naturally by combining movement and mindful eating habits that promote a healthy metabolism.
Prevent and reduce pain, particularly in the joints and lower back, by incorporating gentle stretching and mobility exercises.

Boost your balance and coordination, helping you reduce the risk of falls and injury.

Enhance your overall well-being, physically, mentally, and emotionally, through mindfulness practices and breathing techniques integrated into the yoga routines.

Your Journey Starts Here

This book is an invitation to reclaim your strength, flexibility, and vitality, no matter your age or current fitness level. It's about giving you the tools and guidance you need to thrive well beyond your 60s. By committing to just a few minutes of movement each day, you're investing in yourself, your health, and your independence.

So, why this book? Because you deserve to feel strong, healthy, and confident at every stage of life. This is your time, and this book is your guide.

The Benefits of Staying Active After 60

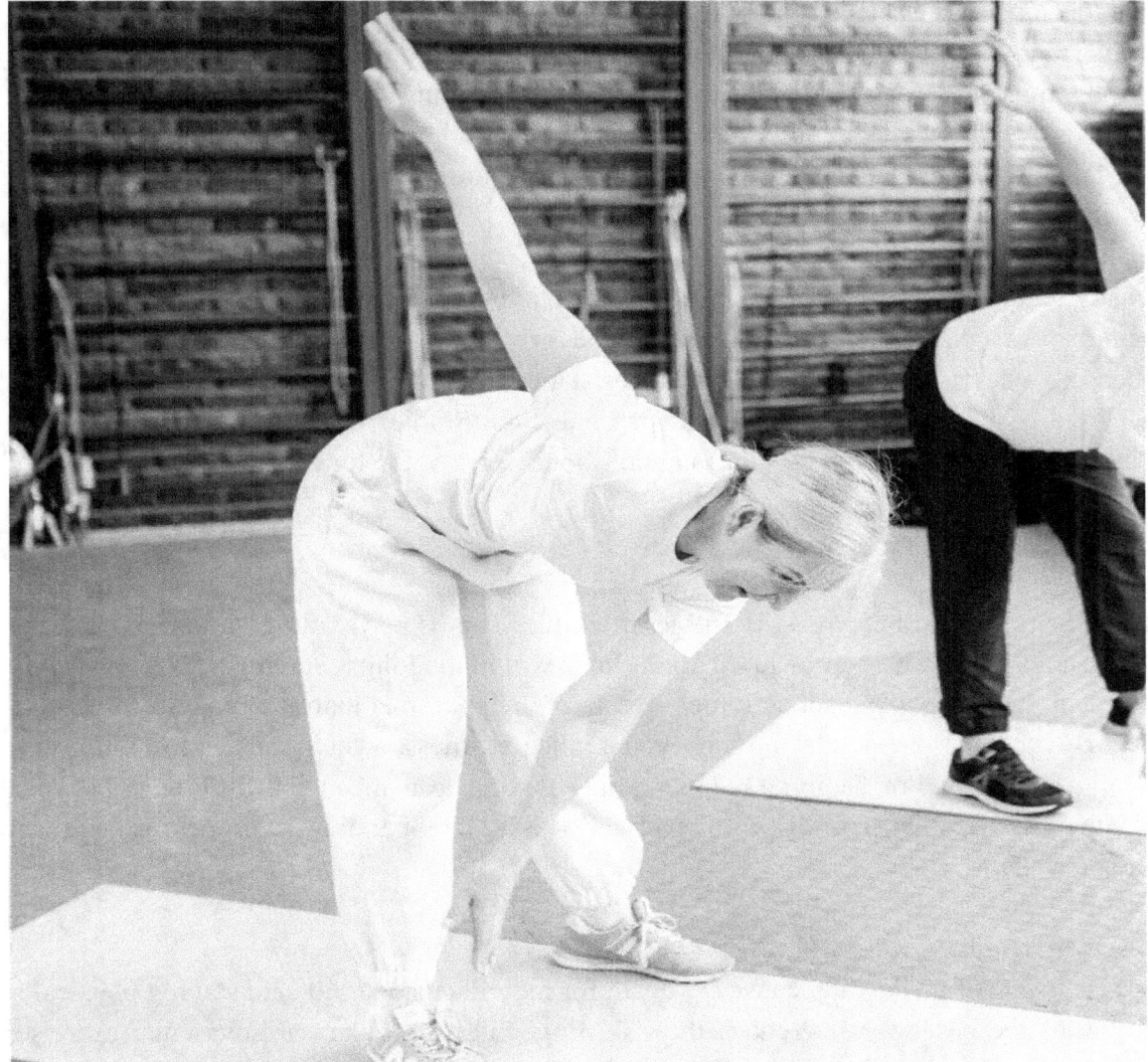

Staying active after 60 is one of the most important things you can do for your body and mind. As we age, it's natural for our bodies to experience changes—slower metabolism, reduced muscle mass, and a decline in bone density. However, these changes don't mean that we have to slow down or stop moving. In fact, staying active becomes even more critical for maintaining health, independence, and overall quality of life. Regular physical activity can be the difference between enjoying your golden years to the fullest or feeling limited by age-related issues.

Physical Benefits of Staying Active After 60

Maintaining Muscle Mass and Strength

One of the most well-known effects of aging is sarcopenia, which is the gradual loss of muscle mass. By the time many individuals reach their 60s and beyond, they may experience a significant decline in muscle strength if they have been inactive. Regular physical activity, particularly strength training, can combat this loss by maintaining or even increasing muscle mass. Strong muscles aren't just for lifting objects or opening jars; they play a key role in balance, posture, and overall mobility. For seniors, maintaining muscle strength means reducing the risk of falls, which can be dangerous as bones become more fragile with age.

Bone Health and Density
Bone density tends to decrease as we age, particularly in post-menopausal women. This can lead to osteoporosis, a condition where bones become brittle and more susceptible to fractures. Weight-bearing exercises, such as walking, resistance training, and even chair yoga, help stimulate bone tissue and slow the process of bone loss. Studies have shown that those who engage in regular physical activity can maintain bone density for longer, reducing the risk of fractures and breaks.

Flexibility and Joint Health
As we age, our joints can become stiff and less flexible. This is partly due to a loss of cartilage and a decrease in the production of lubricating fluids within the joints. Staying active, especially through stretching and low-impact activities like yoga, helps to maintain the range of motion in the joints. By keeping the joints moving, you reduce stiffness, which can lead to improved mobility and less pain. For seniors, keeping joints flexible can mean the difference between moving with ease and struggling with everyday tasks like bending over or reaching for something on a shelf.

Cardiovascular Health
Heart disease is one of the leading causes of death for individuals over 60, and staying physically active is one of the best ways to reduce the risk. Engaging in regular cardiovascular exercise, such as brisk walking, swimming, or even dancing, strengthens the heart and improves circulation. A strong heart pumps blood more efficiently, lowering blood pressure and reducing the risk of heart attacks and strokes. Additionally, cardiovascular exercise helps to manage cholesterol levels, lowering bad cholesterol (LDL) and raising good cholesterol (HDL).

Weight Management and Metabolism
Many people find that as they age, it becomes harder to maintain a healthy weight. This is partly due to a slower metabolism, as the body's ability to burn calories decreases with age. However, regular physical activity can help rev up the metabolism, making it easier to manage weight. Strength training, in particular, is effective for boosting metabolism because muscle tissue burns more calories at rest than fat tissue. For seniors, maintaining a healthy weight is crucial for preventing or managing conditions such as diabetes, hypertension, and cardiovascular disease.

Reducing the Risk of Chronic Diseases

Physical inactivity has been linked to a number of chronic conditions, including type 2 diabetes, heart disease, and certain cancers. Regular exercise, on the other hand, can significantly lower the risk of developing these diseases. For example, aerobic activity helps regulate blood sugar levels, which is key to preventing or managing type 2 diabetes. In addition, exercise has been shown to reduce inflammation in the body, which is linked to many age-related diseases, including Alzheimer's disease.

Mental and Emotional Benefits of Staying Active After 60

Improved Cognitive Function

Cognitive decline is a concern for many seniors, as conditions such as dementia and Alzheimer's disease become more common with age. However, staying physically active can help keep the brain sharp. Studies have found that regular exercise increases blood flow to the brain, which can enhance memory, focus, and problem-solving skills. Physical activity also promotes the growth of new neurons and improves the brain's ability to adapt, a process known as neuroplasticity. Seniors who remain active are more likely to retain cognitive function and delay the onset of cognitive decline.

Enhanced Mood and Mental Health

Exercise is a powerful tool for improving mood and reducing the risk of mental health conditions such as depression and anxiety. Physical activity stimulates the release of endorphins, the body's natural "feel-good" chemicals, which can boost mood and reduce feelings of stress or sadness. Seniors who engage in regular physical activity often report feeling more energetic, positive, and mentally clear. This is particularly important for older adults, who may face isolation, loneliness, or anxiety about aging. Exercise provides a natural outlet for stress relief and fosters a sense of accomplishment and purpose.

Better Sleep

Many seniors struggle with sleep issues, such as insomnia or waking up frequently throughout the night. Regular physical activity can help regulate sleep patterns by promoting deeper, more restful sleep. Exercise helps to tire out the body and reduce feelings of restlessness or anxiety, making it easier to fall asleep and stay asleep. For older adults, a good night's sleep is essential for both physical and mental health. Sleep plays a vital role in the body's healing processes, and it also contributes to better mood and cognitive function.

Increased Social Connections

While many people think of exercise as a solo activity, it can also be a wonderful way to connect with others. Group exercise classes, walking clubs, or even inviting a friend to join you for a chair yoga session can foster a sense of community and reduce feelings of loneliness. For seniors, social connections are just as important as physical health, as they contribute to emotional well-being and reduce the risk of depression. Staying active with others creates opportunities for meaningful interactions and shared experiences, which can enhance quality of life in later years.

Maintaining Independence Through Activity

One of the most significant benefits of staying active after 60 is the ability to maintain independence. As we age, it's common to experience a decline in physical abilities, but regular exercise can slow this decline and keep you functioning at a high level. Activities such as strength training, balance exercises, and flexibility work are key to maintaining mobility and preventing falls. Seniors who stay active are more likely to be able to perform daily tasks independently, such as getting dressed, cooking meals, or going grocery shopping.

For many older adults, the fear of losing independence is a significant concern. Physical activity provides a way to take control of your health and continue living life on your own terms. By staying strong, flexible, and mobile, you reduce the likelihood of needing assistance or moving to a care facility. Instead, you can continue enjoying the activities you love, whether that's gardening, traveling, or playing with your grandchildren.

A Holistic Approach to Staying Active

It's important to remember that staying active doesn't mean engaging in high-intensity workouts or pushing your body to the limit. A balanced approach, incorporating cardiovascular exercise, strength training, flexibility work, and mindfulness practices like yoga, is key to reaping the full benefits of physical activity after 60. Tailoring your exercise routine to your individual needs, limitations, and goals is essential for long-term success.

Activities like chair yoga offer a gentle yet effective way to stay flexible and strong, while strength training helps maintain muscle mass and bone density. Walking or swimming provides cardiovascular benefits without putting too much strain on the joints. Even activities like gardening, dancing, or playing with pets can contribute to staying active and enjoying life to the fullest.

Incorporating mindfulness and relaxation techniques, such as deep breathing or meditation, can further enhance the mental and emotional benefits of physical activity. Mind-body practices like yoga or Tai Chi not only improve flexibility and strength but also promote a sense of calm and well-being.

Staying active after 60 is about more than just exercise—it's about maintaining your independence, supporting your physical and mental health, and enhancing your quality of life. Whether you're new to exercise or a seasoned fitness enthusiast, it's never too late to start moving. The benefits of regular physical activity are undeniable, and with the right approach, you can enjoy a healthy, active, and fulfilling life well into your later years.

A Holistic Approach: Weight Loss, Strength, and Flexibility

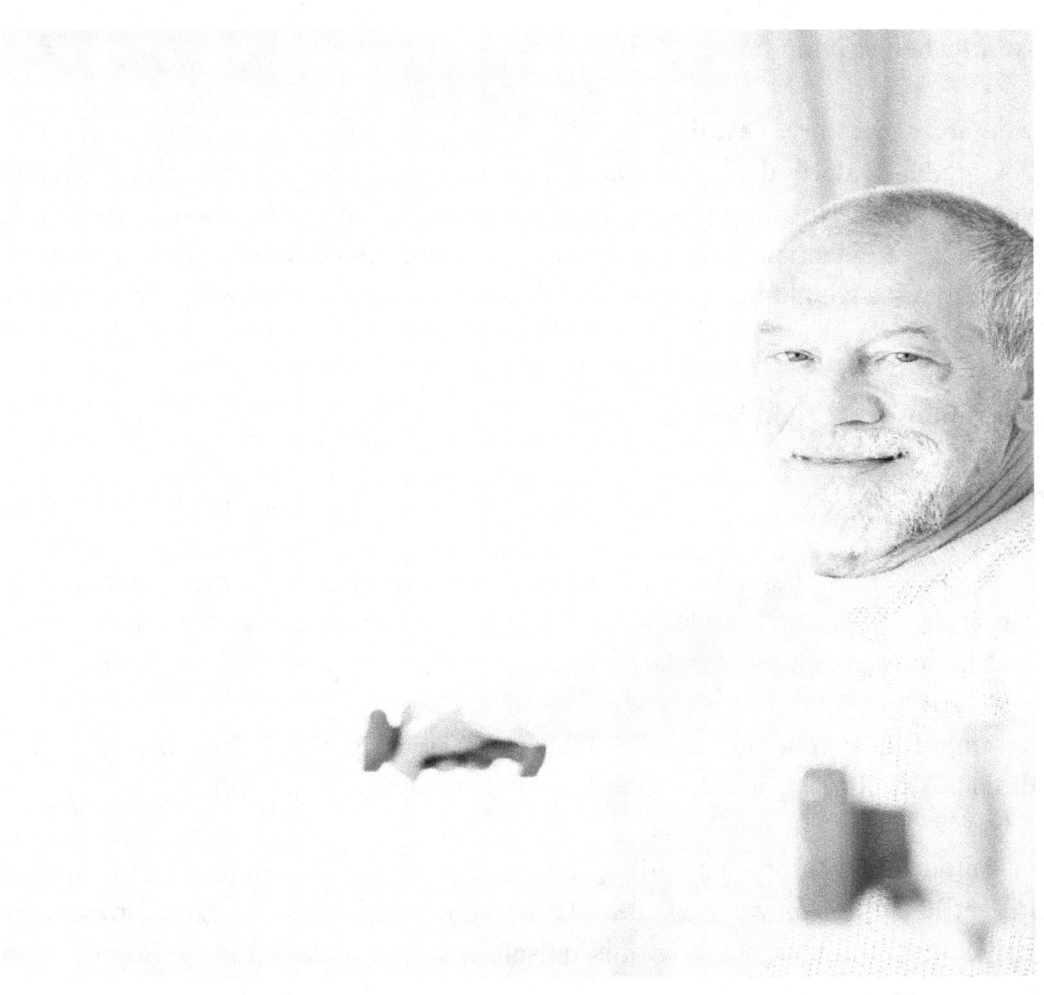

As we age, maintaining health and mobility becomes increasingly important, but the way we approach fitness must evolve as well. No longer can we rely on the same high-intensity routines of our younger years. Instead, it's essential to adopt a more thoughtful, balanced approach that integrates all aspects of well-being. A holistic fitness routine is key to living a fuller, more active life after 60. This approach combines three essential pillars: weight loss, strength, and flexibility.

When approached thoughtfully, these elements work together to improve overall quality of life, reduce pain, increase vitality, and, most importantly, keep us independent for as long as possible.

Let's break down what each component entails and how they intertwine to create a balanced, sustainable fitness routine for seniors.

Weight Loss: The Foundation of Physical Wellness
For many people over 60, weight loss isn't just about looking good—it's about feeling good. As metabolism slows down with age, it becomes easier to gain weight, particularly around the midsection. This extra weight can exacerbate issues like joint pain, high blood pressure, and diabetes. However, weight loss in seniors must be approached carefully. Dramatic, unsustainable weight loss can lead to muscle loss, frailty, and nutritional deficiencies, which is the opposite of what we want when striving for long-term health.

To lose weight in a healthy way, the key is combining mindful eating with gentle but consistent exercise. A gradual calorie deficit—created through diet and activity—is more sustainable than aggressive crash diets. Nutrition plays a huge role here: diets rich in lean protein, whole grains, and healthy fats are essential. But exercise is equally important. While burning calories through physical activity aids weight loss, it also helps maintain muscle mass, which is crucial to keeping metabolism steady.

Key considerations for weight loss in seniors:

Start slow and steady: Focus on small, achievable goals that prioritize gradual fat loss while preserving muscle.
Create a calorie deficit: Pair mild to moderate exercise with a balanced diet. Avoid cutting calories too drastically, as this can lead to nutrient deficiencies and muscle loss.
Hydrate: Drinking enough water is crucial for digestion, energy, and maintaining muscle function.
Prioritize protein: Protein helps maintain muscle mass during weight loss and supports recovery after workouts. Aim for lean sources like fish, chicken, legumes, and tofu.
Strength: The Engine of Independence
Strength is about much more than lifting heavy objects. It's the engine that keeps your body functioning efficiently. As we age, muscle mass naturally decreases, a process known as sarcopenia. Without strength training, this muscle loss can lead to frailty, loss of balance, and increased risk of falls—one of the biggest threats to seniors' independence. Strength also plays a pivotal role in boosting metabolism, even while at rest, which aids in weight management.

The beauty of strength training is that it doesn't have to be extreme to be effective. For seniors, even light resistance training, done consistently, can yield significant benefits. Exercises using your body weight or light dumbbells can improve muscle tone, balance, and functional strength. Functional strength refers to the type of strength you need for everyday activities—standing up from a chair, lifting groceries, or climbing stairs. These movements, when reinforced through regular strength training, reduce the risk of injury and allow seniors to live more independently.

Why strength matters for seniors:

Improved mobility and balance: Strength training enhances coordination, helping prevent falls—a major cause of injury for seniors.
Preserving muscle mass: As muscle mass decreases with age, strength training is essential to prevent muscle wasting, which can severely limit daily activity.
Increased bone density: Strength training puts stress on the bones, which in turn stimulates them to become denser, reducing the risk of osteoporosis and fractures.
Better metabolic health: Building and maintaining muscle boosts your metabolism, helping with weight control and improving blood sugar regulation, particularly important for managing or preventing type 2 diabetes.
Exercises to build strength for seniors:

Chair-assisted squats: These squats, done while holding onto a chair, build leg strength without putting undue pressure on the knees or lower back.
Seated leg lifts: A simple exercise to engage your hip flexors and abdominal muscles.
Seated bicep curls: Using light weights, this exercise strengthens the arms, making daily tasks like lifting and carrying easier.
Overhead presses: Using light weights or resistance bands, this movement strengthens your shoulders and upper arms, essential for reaching overhead or pushing up from a seated position.
Bodyweight exercises: From modified push-ups to wall planks, bodyweight exercises can significantly improve muscle tone, especially when combined with chair-based movements for additional support.
Flexibility: The Secret to Pain-Free Movement
Flexibility is often an overlooked component of fitness, but it's crucial for maintaining pain-free movement and overall mobility. As the body ages, connective tissues like tendons and ligaments lose elasticity, making muscles tighter and joints stiffer. This can lead to a restricted range of motion, poor posture, and chronic pain, particularly in the lower back, shoulders, and hips. Incorporating flexibility exercises into your routine can help counteract these issues, ensuring that you move more freely and with less discomfort.

Flexibility exercises for seniors should be slow, controlled, and mindful. Stretching before and after workouts helps prevent injury and eases stiffness. Chair yoga, in particular, offers a gentle, effective way to increase flexibility while improving balance and posture. Chair yoga eliminates the need for getting down on the floor, making it ideal for seniors who may have mobility issues.

Benefits of flexibility exercises for seniors:

Pain reduction: Regular stretching can alleviate chronic pain in the joints and muscles by releasing tension and improving circulation.

Improved posture: Flexibility helps align the body, reducing strain on muscles and joints and preventing the hunched posture many seniors develop over time.

Enhanced balance: Increased flexibility improves body awareness, allowing for better balance and reducing the risk of falls.

Greater ease in daily activities: Simple tasks like bending over, reaching for objects, or even walking become easier when your body is flexible and limber.

Effective flexibility exercises for seniors:

Seated hamstring stretch: While seated on a chair, gently reach toward your toes to stretch the back of your legs and lower back.

Neck stretches: Slowly tilt your head from side to side to relieve neck tension and improve mobility.

Seated spinal twists: While sitting upright, twist your torso gently to each side to stretch the lower back and spine.

Chest and shoulder openers: These stretches help counteract the hunching posture common in seniors, relieving tightness in the chest and improving shoulder mobility.

Hip flexor stretches: Keeping your hips flexible is essential for walking, bending, and standing. Seated or standing hip flexor stretches help maintain this important range of motion.

How They Work Together

What makes a holistic approach so powerful is the way these three components—weight loss, strength, and flexibility—work together to amplify results. Strength training helps with weight loss by preserving muscle mass and increasing metabolism. Flexibility exercises, in turn, support strength training by improving range of motion and reducing the risk of injury. Weight loss reduces strain on joints, making flexibility and strength training exercises easier and less painful. When you combine all three in a balanced routine, you're setting yourself up for long-term success.

Here's how you can integrate all three in your fitness plan:

Start with flexibility: Begin each session with gentle stretching or chair yoga to loosen up your muscles and joints, preparing your body for movement.

Move into strength training: After stretching, engage in light strength exercises. Focus on major muscle groups to build functional strength.

Finish with cardio or gentle movement: If weight loss is your goal, finish your routine with a short period of low-impact cardio, like walking or light cycling, to burn extra calories.

By embracing this holistic approach, you're not only exercising to look or feel better—you're investing in your ability to move freely, confidently, and without pain for years to come. The key is consistency. Make weight loss, strength, and flexibility a regular part of your routine, and you'll experience an overall sense of well-being that goes beyond just physical fitness.

Chair Yoga and Strength Training: A Perfect Combination

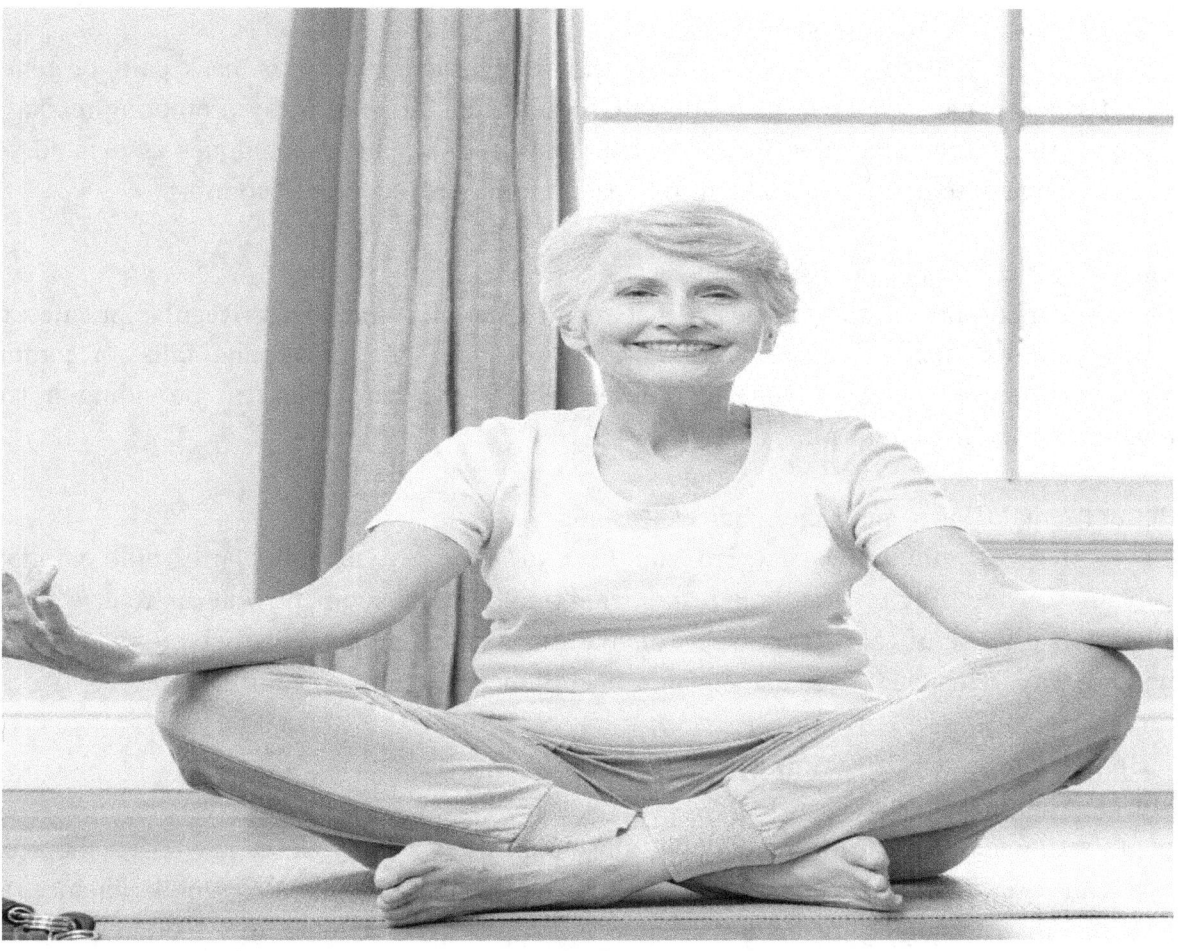

As we age, maintaining our health and mobility becomes increasingly important. For seniors, finding suitable forms of exercise that promote flexibility, strength, and overall well-being is essential. Enter chair yoga and strength training—a powerful combination that caters to the needs of seniors, allowing them to exercise safely and effectively from the comfort of their own homes. This chapter will explore the benefits of chair yoga and strength training, how they complement each other, and provide you with practical exercises and routines to incorporate into your daily life.

The Benefits of Chair Yoga

1. Enhanced Flexibility

Chair yoga is a gentle form of yoga that allows individuals to perform stretches and poses while seated, making it accessible for those with limited mobility. One of the primary benefits of chair yoga is improved flexibility. As we age, our muscles and joints can become stiffer, leading to a decreased range of motion. Regular practice of chair yoga can help counteract this stiffness, making everyday activities easier and more comfortable.

2. Reduced Pain and Discomfort

Many seniors experience chronic pain due to conditions such as arthritis, back pain, or general muscle tension. Chair yoga can help alleviate some of this discomfort by promoting relaxation and gentle stretching. The mindful movements and deep breathing techniques associated with yoga can also help reduce stress and tension, leading to improved overall comfort.

3. Improved Balance and Coordination

Chair yoga incorporates various poses that require stability and focus. Regular practice can enhance your balance and coordination, which are crucial for preventing falls—a common concern for seniors. Many chair yoga poses engage the core muscles, providing a solid foundation for maintaining balance.

4. Better Mental Clarity and Emotional Well-Being

Yoga emphasizes mindfulness, which can lead to improved mental clarity and emotional well-being. By focusing on your breath and being present in the moment, you can reduce anxiety and promote a sense of calm. This aspect of chair yoga is particularly beneficial for seniors, as it provides a way to manage stress and enhance overall mental health.

The Benefits of Strength Training

1. Muscle Maintenance and Growth

Strength training is crucial for maintaining muscle mass, especially as we age. After the age of 30, we can lose 3-5% of our muscle mass per decade, which can impact strength, balance, and overall mobility. Engaging in regular strength training helps counteract this decline, promoting muscle maintenance and even growth.

2. Increased Bone Density

Strength training is not only beneficial for muscles but also for bones. Weight-bearing exercises help stimulate bone growth and increase bone density, reducing the risk of osteoporosis and fractures. This is especially important for women over 60, who are at a higher risk for bone density loss.

3. Enhanced Functional Fitness
Strength training improves functional fitness, which is the ability to perform everyday activities with ease and confidence. By incorporating strength exercises into your routine, you can make tasks like lifting groceries, climbing stairs, and even getting out of a chair easier and safer.

4. Boosted Metabolism and Weight Management
As muscle mass increases, so does your resting metabolic rate, meaning you burn more calories at rest. This is particularly important for seniors looking to manage their weight. Combined with chair yoga, which encourages mindful eating and healthy lifestyle choices, strength training can contribute significantly to overall weight management.

The Perfect Combination: Chair Yoga and Strength Training
While both chair yoga and strength training offer numerous benefits on their own, together they create a balanced fitness routine tailored to the needs of seniors. Here's why combining these two forms of exercise is particularly effective:

1. Comprehensive Approach to Fitness
Combining chair yoga and strength training provides a comprehensive approach to fitness, addressing flexibility, strength, balance, and mental well-being. While chair yoga improves flexibility and relaxation, strength training builds muscle and promotes stability. Together, they create a well-rounded program that supports overall health.

2. Adaptability and Accessibility
Both chair yoga and strength training can be easily adapted to meet individual fitness levels and limitations. Whether you're a beginner or more experienced, you can modify exercises to suit your needs. This adaptability ensures that seniors of all fitness levels can participate safely and effectively.

3. Enhanced Recovery and Injury Prevention
Chair yoga can be an excellent complement to strength training, aiding in recovery and injury prevention. After a strength training session, gentle stretching and relaxation through chair yoga can help alleviate muscle soreness and stiffness, promoting faster recovery. Furthermore, improved flexibility and balance can reduce the risk of injuries during strength exercises.

4. Mind-Body Connection
The mindfulness inherent in yoga fosters a deeper awareness of your body, which can enhance your strength training experience. As you engage in strength exercises, this heightened

awareness allows you to focus on proper form and alignment, reducing the risk of injury and maximizing the benefits of each movement.

Practical Exercises: Chair Yoga and Strength Training Routine
Now that we've established the benefits of chair yoga and strength training, let's look at some practical exercises you can incorporate into your routine. Aim for at least 30 minutes of combined exercise several times a week. You can start with chair yoga for 15 minutes, followed by strength training for 15 minutes.

Chair Yoga Poses
Seated Cat-Cow Stretch

Sit tall in your chair with feet flat on the floor.
Inhale as you arch your back and look up (Cow Pose).
Exhale as you round your back and tuck your chin (Cat Pose).
Repeat 5-10 times.
Seated Forward Bend

Sit at the edge of your chair, feet hip-width apart.
Inhale and reach your arms overhead.
Exhale and hinge at your hips, reaching toward the floor.
Hold for 5 breaths, feeling the stretch in your back and hamstrings.
Seated Twist

Sit tall with feet flat.
Inhale and lengthen your spine, then exhale as you twist to one side, using the chair for support.
Hold for 5 breaths, then repeat on the other side.

Seated Side Stretch

Sit tall and reach one arm overhead.
Lean to the opposite side, feeling the stretch along your side body.
Hold for 5 breaths, then switch sides.
Strength Training Exercises
Seated Leg Lifts

Sit tall in your chair with your feet flat.
Extend one leg straight out in front of you, keeping your knee straight.
Hold for a few seconds, then lower back down. Repeat 10-15 times on each leg.
Chair-Assisted Squats

Stand in front of your chair with feet shoulder-width apart.
Lower your body as if you're going to sit down, stopping just above the seat.
Stand back up and repeat for 10-15 repetitions.

Seated Bicep Curls

Sit tall with a light weight in each hand (or use water bottles).
Keep your elbows close to your body and curl the weights towards your shoulders.
Lower back down slowly. Repeat for 10-15 repetitions.

Overhead Press

Sit tall with a weight in each hand.
Raise the weights above your head, keeping your core engaged.
Lower back down to shoulder height and repeat for 10-15 repetitions.
Creating a Routine
Here's a simple routine you can follow:

Warm-Up (5 minutes)

Gentle neck rolls, shoulder rolls, and wrist rotations.
Chair Yoga (15 minutes)

Seated Cat-Cow Stretch: 5-10 repetitions.
Seated Forward Bend: Hold for 5 breaths.
Seated Twist: Hold for 5 breaths on each side.
Seated Side Stretch: Hold for 5 breaths on each side.
Strength Training (15 minutes)

Seated Leg Lifts: 10-15 repetitions per leg.
Chair-Assisted Squats: 10-15 repetitions.
Seated Bicep Curls: 10-15 repetitions.
Overhead Press: 10-15 repetitions.
Cool Down (5 minutes)

Gentle seated stretches, focusing on the breath.

Chair yoga and strength training are a perfect combination for seniors seeking to enhance their health and well-being. By embracing these practices, you can improve your flexibility, build strength, and foster a greater sense of mental clarity and emotional balance. Remember, the journey to better health is not just about the exercises you do, but also about the lifestyle changes you embrace along the way. So take a deep breath, sit tall in your chair, and embark on this journey toward a healthier, more active life.

Chapter 1: The Power of Gentle Movement

How Exercise Enhances Longevity and Well-being

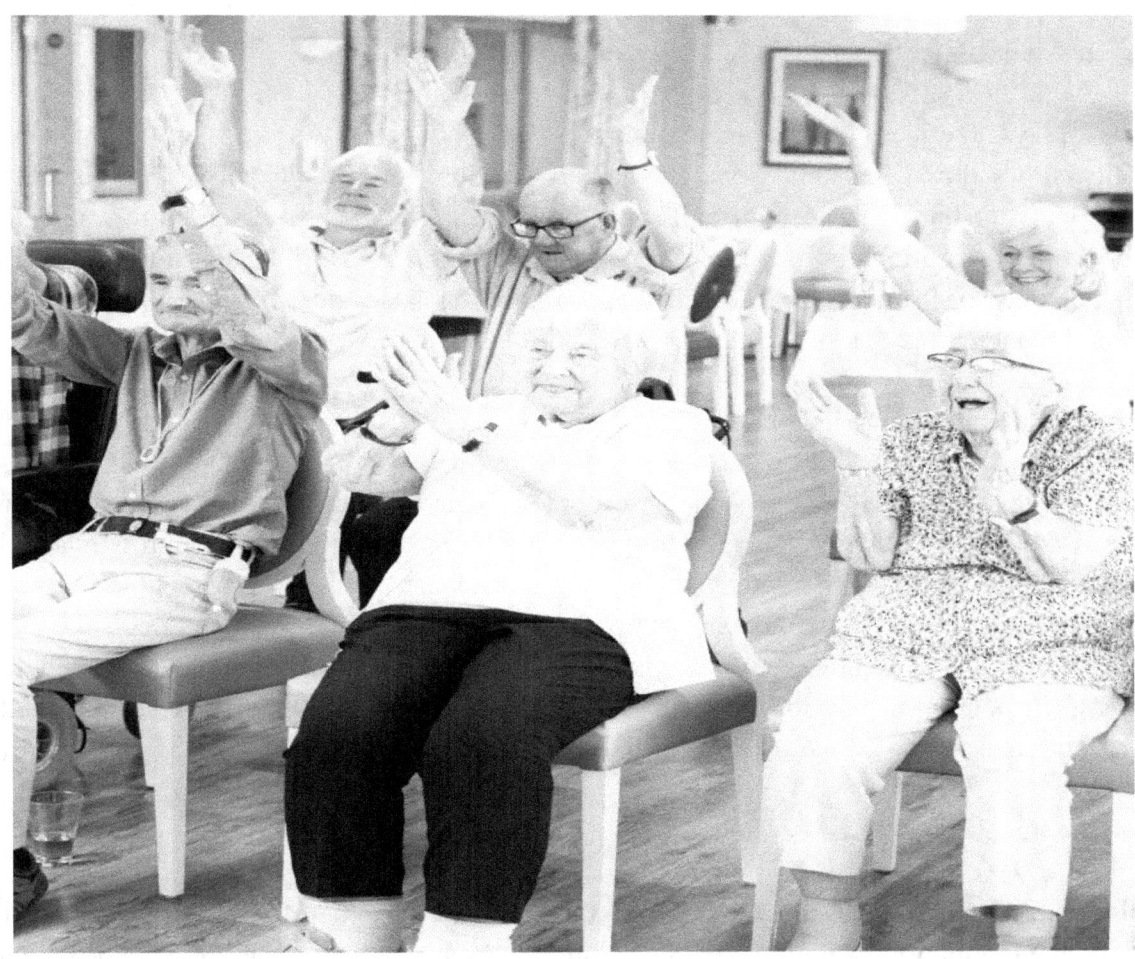

Exercise is often touted as a cornerstone of a healthy lifestyle, especially for seniors. Engaging in regular physical activity can profoundly influence longevity and overall well-being. But how exactly does exercise affect our bodies and minds as we age? Let's delve into the intricate relationship between exercise and a longer, healthier life, exploring its physiological benefits, psychological effects, and the various forms of exercise that contribute to enhanced vitality.

The Physiological Benefits of Exercise
1. Cardiovascular Health

One of the most significant benefits of exercise is its positive impact on cardiovascular health. Regular physical activity strengthens the heart muscle, improving its efficiency in pumping blood. This enhanced blood flow ensures that oxygen and nutrients reach vital organs and tissues more effectively, reducing the risk of heart disease, hypertension, and stroke. According to the American Heart Association, engaging in moderate aerobic exercise for at least 150 minutes weekly can dramatically lower the risk of cardiovascular-related conditions.

2. Weight Management

Exercise plays a crucial role in maintaining a healthy weight. As we age, our metabolism naturally slows down, leading to weight gain if we don't adjust our activity levels. Regular exercise helps to burn calories and build lean muscle mass, which is essential for maintaining metabolic rate. Additionally, incorporating strength training can further enhance muscle mass, which not only contributes to a healthier appearance but also aids in regulating blood sugar levels and reducing the risk of type 2 diabetes.

3. Bone Density and Joint Health

Another critical aspect of aging is the loss of bone density and joint health. Weight-bearing exercises, such as walking, dancing, or strength training, stimulate bone growth and help maintain bone density, significantly reducing the risk of osteoporosis and fractures. Moreover, exercise promotes joint flexibility and strength, alleviating stiffness and reducing the risk of arthritis-related pain. Gentle activities like yoga and tai chi can be particularly beneficial, providing a low-impact way to strengthen muscles and improve balance, which is essential for fall prevention.

4. Immune Function

Regular exercise has been shown to boost the immune system. Moderate physical activity increases the circulation of immune cells, making the body more adept at combating infections. Moreover, it helps reduce inflammation, a key factor in many chronic diseases associated with aging. By engaging in regular exercise, seniors can enhance their immune response, allowing them to better fend off illness and maintain overall health.

5. Cognitive Function

Physical activity is not just beneficial for the body; it has profound effects on brain health. Studies indicate that regular exercise can slow the cognitive decline often associated with aging. Exercise promotes the release of brain-derived neurotrophic factor (BDNF), a protein that supports the growth and survival of neurons. This leads to improvements in memory, attention, and overall cognitive function. Aerobic activities, in particular, have been linked to enhanced brain health, reducing the risk of conditions like Alzheimer's disease and other forms of dementia.

The Psychological Effects of Exercise
1. Mood Enhancement

Exercise has a well-documented effect on mental health. When you engage in physical activity, your body releases endorphins, often referred to as "feel-good" hormones. These natural chemicals act as mood lifters and can help alleviate symptoms of depression and anxiety. For seniors, who may experience feelings of isolation or loneliness, regular physical activity can serve as a vital outlet for improving mood and emotional well-being.

2. Stress Reduction

In addition to mood enhancement, exercise is a powerful stress reliever. Engaging in physical activity reduces levels of the body's stress hormones, such as adrenaline and cortisol. This reduction can lead to a significant decrease in feelings of stress and anxiety. Mind-body exercises, like yoga and tai chi, combine movement with breathing techniques and meditation, providing an added layer of relaxation and mindfulness that further helps to manage stress.

3. Improved Sleep Quality

Regular exercise can also lead to better sleep quality. Many seniors struggle with insomnia or disrupted sleep patterns, which can significantly impact overall health and quality of life. Engaging in physical activity, particularly earlier in the day, can help regulate sleep patterns, allowing for deeper and more restorative sleep. Improved sleep enhances mood, cognitive function, and energy levels, creating a positive feedback loop that encourages further physical activity.

4. Enhanced Social Interaction

For many seniors, exercise provides an opportunity for social interaction. Joining exercise classes, walking groups, or community fitness programs fosters connections with others, combating feelings of loneliness and isolation. Social engagement is crucial for mental well-being, providing emotional support and a sense of belonging. The bonds formed through shared physical activity can lead to lasting friendships and a more fulfilling life.

Finding the Right Exercise

With all these benefits in mind, it's essential to understand that not all exercise needs to be intense or time-consuming to be effective. The key is finding enjoyable activities that fit into your lifestyle. Here are some recommendations for incorporating exercise into your daily routine:

1. Aerobic Activities

Walking, swimming, cycling, or dancing are excellent low-impact options that can be easily adapted to your fitness level. Aim for at least 150 minutes of moderate-intensity aerobic activity per week, breaking it into manageable sessions.

2. Strength Training

Incorporate strength training exercises at least twice a week. Use light weights, resistance bands, or even bodyweight exercises like squats and lunges to build muscle and improve overall strength. Focus on major muscle groups to enhance functional fitness.

3. Flexibility and Balance Exercises

Incorporate stretching routines, yoga, or tai chi to improve flexibility and balance. These activities not only enhance physical capabilities but also promote relaxation and mental clarity.

4. Make it Social

Engage in group classes, exercise with a friend, or join community programs. The social aspect of exercise can enhance motivation and adherence to your routine.

Exercise is a vital component of longevity and well-being, particularly for seniors. The physiological benefits, including improved cardiovascular health, weight management, and cognitive function, complement the psychological advantages such as enhanced mood and stress relief. By incorporating a variety of physical activities into your routine, you can not only extend your lifespan but also improve the quality of your life, enabling you to enjoy each day with vitality and purpose. Embrace the power of movement—your body and mind will thank you.

Common Exercise Myths for Seniors

As a fitness instructor and exercise expert, I've encountered numerous misconceptions about exercise, especially concerning seniors. Understanding and dispelling these myths is crucial for promoting a healthy lifestyle among older adults. Let's dive into some of the most prevalent exercise myths and clarify the truths behind them.

Myth 1: Seniors Should Avoid Exercise to Prevent Injury
Truth: While it's true that injuries can occur, the idea that seniors should avoid exercise altogether is misguided. In fact, regular physical activity is one of the best ways to enhance strength, balance, and flexibility, all of which contribute to reducing the risk of falls and injuries.

As we age, our muscles and bones naturally weaken, leading to an increased risk of falls. Engaging in a consistent exercise program can help counteract this process. Activities like strength training, yoga, and balance exercises can strengthen muscles, improve coordination, and enhance overall stability. It's essential to choose low-impact activities and to consult with a healthcare provider before starting any new exercise routine.

Myth 2: All Seniors Are Too Frail for Strength Training
Truth: Many seniors believe that lifting weights or performing resistance exercises is only for younger individuals or those who are already fit. This myth is harmful, as strength training is incredibly beneficial for seniors and can be adapted to suit various fitness levels.

Research shows that strength training can lead to significant improvements in muscle mass, bone density, and functional ability. Even individuals who are frail or have chronic conditions can engage in modified strength training. Using resistance bands, light dumbbells, or even body-weight exercises like squats and modified push-ups can provide substantial benefits.

Myth 3: Stretching is Only for Athletes
Truth: Stretching is often perceived as a practice reserved for athletes, but this misconception overlooks its essential role in maintaining flexibility and mobility for everyone, particularly seniors.

As we age, our muscles and joints become stiffer, leading to decreased range of motion. Incorporating stretching into your daily routine can help counteract this stiffness, reduce the risk of injury, and alleviate muscle tension. Simple stretches, such as seated hamstring stretches or gentle shoulder rolls, can be performed in a chair and are accessible for most seniors.

Myth 4: Exercise is Not Necessary if I Have a Sedentary Lifestyle
Truth: Some seniors believe that they can skip exercise if they feel generally healthy or active in their daily routines. However, the truth is that exercise is essential for everyone, regardless of their lifestyle.

While daily activities like walking, gardening, or light housework are beneficial, they often don't provide the structured exercise needed to improve cardiovascular health, strength, and flexibility. Seniors should aim for a balanced routine that includes aerobic, strength, flexibility, and balance exercises to enhance their overall well-being. Even short bouts of activity can lead to significant health improvements.

Myth 5: Yoga is Only for Young, Flexible People
Truth: Many seniors dismiss yoga because they believe it requires a high level of flexibility or fitness. This myth could not be further from the truth!

Chair yoga, in particular, is an excellent option for seniors who may find traditional yoga poses challenging. It allows individuals to enjoy the benefits of yoga—such as improved flexibility, reduced stress, and enhanced balance—without needing to get on the floor. Many yoga poses can be modified for seniors, making it accessible to everyone, regardless of their initial fitness level.

Myth 6: You Need a Gym to Exercise Effectively
Truth: The notion that effective exercise can only be done in a gym is a significant barrier for many seniors. However, countless exercises can be performed in the comfort of your own home without any specialized equipment.

Chair-based exercises, body-weight movements, and resistance bands are excellent tools for creating an effective home workout routine. Moreover, activities like walking, gardening, or even dancing can contribute significantly to your fitness goals. The key is to find enjoyable activities that promote regular movement.

Myth 7: Older Adults Cannot Recover from Intense Workouts
Truth: While it's true that recovery may take longer as we age, the idea that older adults cannot recover from exercise is misleading. In fact, engaging in regular physical activity can improve recovery times by enhancing blood circulation and promoting muscle repair.

It's important to listen to your body and allow adequate recovery time between workouts. Seniors can benefit from incorporating rest days, staying hydrated, and ensuring proper nutrition to support their recovery. Tailoring exercise intensity to your fitness level is crucial, but with appropriate pacing and modifications, seniors can recover effectively from various workouts.

Myth 8: High-Impact Activities are the Best for Weight Loss
Truth: Many believe that high-impact workouts, such as running or high-intensity interval training (HIIT), are the most effective for weight loss. However, these workouts can be tough on older joints and may not be suitable for everyone.

Low-impact activities, such as walking, swimming, cycling, and chair exercises, can also promote weight loss and improve cardiovascular health without placing excessive stress on the body. Combining aerobic exercises with strength training and flexibility work can create a balanced and effective weight loss plan that is safe and sustainable.

Myth 9: You Need to Exercise for Hours Each Day to See Benefits
Truth: Some seniors feel overwhelmed by the idea that they must commit to lengthy workouts to experience health benefits. The reality is that even short bursts of activity can be effective.

Research indicates that breaking exercise into manageable segments—such as 10 to 15 minutes at a time—can still yield significant health benefits. Consistency is key. Incorporating movement into your daily routine, even in small doses, contributes to overall fitness and wellness.

Myth 10: Exercise Will Make Me Sore or Tired
Truth: While some may experience mild soreness after starting a new exercise routine, the belief that exercise will inevitably lead to fatigue or pain is a common myth. Regular physical activity can enhance energy levels, improve mood, and increase stamina over time.

It's important to ease into new exercises, listen to your body, and choose activities that feel good for you. Over time, as you build strength and endurance, you'll likely find that you have more energy and resilience than before.

Debunking these common exercise myths for seniors is vital for promoting a healthier, more active lifestyle. By understanding the truths behind these misconceptions, seniors can approach exercise with confidence, knowing that movement is not only beneficial but essential for maintaining overall health and well-being.

Embracing regular physical activity tailored to individual needs and abilities can lead to a more fulfilling, active, and independent life. Whether through chair yoga, strength training, or simple stretches, the key is to find joy in movement and remain committed to lifelong health.

The Impact of Chair Yoga on Flexibility and Pain Relief

As we age, maintaining flexibility and managing pain become increasingly essential for overall well-being. For many seniors, traditional forms of exercise may not be feasible due to mobility limitations or chronic conditions. This is where chair yoga emerges as a transformative practice that offers a multitude of benefits, particularly in enhancing flexibility and alleviating pain. This chapter will delve into the profound impact chair yoga can have on seniors, backed by research, personal anecdotes, and practical tips for incorporating this gentle form of exercise into daily routines.

Understanding Chair Yoga

Chair yoga is a modified form of yoga that adapts traditional poses to be performed while seated or using a chair for support. This makes it accessible for individuals with limited mobility, balance issues, or those who may not be comfortable on the floor. Unlike traditional yoga, which often requires a mat and the ability to get up and down, chair yoga allows practitioners to engage in a mindful movement practice without the risk of falling or injury.

The Essence of Chair Yoga

At its core, chair yoga is about promoting the mind-body connection. The practice emphasizes controlled movements, deep breathing, and mindfulness. Each pose is designed to stretch and strengthen muscles, improve posture, and enhance joint flexibility, all of which are crucial for seniors. Additionally, the slow and deliberate nature of chair yoga allows participants to focus on their bodies, cultivating a sense of awareness and presence that can be calming and therapeutic.

Enhancing Flexibility

The Science of Flexibility

Flexibility refers to the range of motion in our joints and muscles. As we age, our bodies naturally lose elasticity, making it harder to perform daily activities like reaching for items on a high shelf or bending down to tie shoes. According to a study published in the Journal of Aging and Physical Activity, regular stretching and flexibility exercises can significantly improve mobility and overall physical function in older adults.

Chair Yoga Poses for Flexibility

Chair yoga offers a variety of poses specifically designed to improve flexibility in different muscle groups. Here are some key poses that can make a significant difference:

Seated Forward Bend: This pose stretches the spine and hamstrings. Sit tall in your chair, inhale deeply, and as you exhale, lean forward gently, allowing your hands to reach toward your feet. This stretch helps elongate the spine and opens up the lower back.

Seated Cat-Cow Stretch: This is a gentle way to enhance spinal flexibility. While seated, alternate between arching your back (cat) and lifting your chest (cow) as you breathe in and out. This movement promotes better spinal mobility and can alleviate tension in the back.

Gentle Side Stretches: Sitting tall, raise one arm overhead and lean to the opposite side, stretching the side of your body. Alternate sides to promote flexibility in the obliques and intercostal muscles, which can improve overall torso mobility.

Seated Hip Openers: Cross one ankle over the opposite knee and gently press down on the raised knee. This pose helps to open the hips, an area that can become tight with age.

Seated Twist: Place your right hand on the back of your chair and twist to the right, looking over your shoulder. This pose enhances spinal flexibility and aids digestion, making it a great addition to your routine.

Long-Term Flexibility Benefits
Regular practice of these chair yoga poses can lead to lasting improvements in flexibility. Enhanced flexibility not only allows for easier movement in daily activities but also reduces the risk of injury. Improved range of motion can alleviate stiffness, making it easier to engage in social activities, hobbies, or even household chores.

Alleviating Pain
Understanding Pain in Seniors
Chronic pain is a common issue for seniors, often stemming from conditions like arthritis, fibromyalgia, or general wear and tear on the body. According to the National Institute of Health, approximately 50% of older adults report experiencing chronic pain, which can severely impact their quality of life. Pain can lead to decreased mobility, increased reliance on medications, and reduced overall activity levels.

The Role of Chair Yoga in Pain Management
Chair yoga addresses pain on multiple fronts. Firstly, the gentle movements involved in chair yoga help to increase blood flow and circulation, which can alleviate stiffness and discomfort in the joints and muscles. Secondly, the mindfulness aspect of yoga encourages relaxation and stress reduction, which are crucial for pain management. Stress can exacerbate pain levels, creating a vicious cycle that's hard to break.

Techniques to Alleviate Pain Through Chair Yoga
Here are specific chair yoga techniques aimed at pain relief:

Deep Breathing Exercises: Incorporate deep breathing at the beginning and end of your session. Inhale deeply through your nose, filling your abdomen, and exhale slowly through your mouth. This practice calms the nervous system and reduces overall stress, which can lower perceived pain levels.

Gentle Neck Rolls: As tension often builds in the neck and shoulders, gentle neck rolls can relieve this discomfort. Slowly roll your head in a circular motion, allowing your neck to release tension while focusing on your breath.

Wrist and Finger Stretches: Many seniors experience pain in their hands and wrists due to arthritis. Gentle wrist circles and finger stretches can enhance circulation and reduce stiffness, making daily tasks more manageable.

Chair Pigeon Pose: This pose is excellent for relieving hip pain. While seated, place one ankle on the opposite knee and gently press down on the knee. This opens up the hips and alleviates tension in the lower back.

Relaxation Pose: After your practice, spend a few moments in a seated relaxation pose. Sit back in your chair with your hands on your thighs, close your eyes, and focus on your breath. This time of relaxation allows the body to absorb the benefits of the exercises while promoting a sense of peace.

Research Supporting Pain Relief
A growing body of research supports the effectiveness of yoga in alleviating chronic pain. A study published in the Journal of Pain Research found that participants who practiced yoga reported significant reductions in pain and improvements in overall quality of life. The gentle nature of chair yoga makes it a suitable alternative for those who may not tolerate more vigorous forms of exercise.

Creating a Chair Yoga Routine
How to Get Started
Starting a chair yoga routine is easy and can be done from the comfort of your own home. Here are steps to help you get started:

Choose a Comfortable Chair: Select a sturdy chair without arms that allows you to sit with your feet flat on the ground.

Set a Regular Schedule: Aim for at least 20-30 minutes of practice a few times a week. Consistency is key to experiencing the benefits.

Follow Guided Sessions: If you're new to chair yoga, consider following online classes or video tutorials that guide you through the poses and breathing techniques.

Listen to Your Body: Pay attention to how your body feels during each pose. If something doesn't feel right, modify the pose or skip it altogether.

Invite Others: Practicing with friends or family can make the experience more enjoyable and provide motivation.

The impact of chair yoga on flexibility and pain relief for seniors is profound and multifaceted. This gentle yet effective practice allows older adults to enhance their physical abilities while fostering a sense of calm and well-being. By integrating chair yoga into daily routines, seniors can reclaim their mobility, reduce pain levels, and significantly improve their overall quality of life. With the right mindset and a commitment to regular practice, the journey toward better flexibility and pain management can begin right from the comfort of one's chair.

Strength Training for Everyday Functionality

Strength training is not just about building muscles or achieving a sculpted physique; it's about enhancing your ability to perform everyday activities with ease and confidence. For seniors, especially those over 60, strength training offers a plethora of benefits that go beyond aesthetics. It can improve balance, enhance mobility, increase bone density, and even contribute to better mental health. This chapter delves into the importance of strength training for everyday functionality, how it can be safely incorporated into your routine, and specific exercises tailored for seniors.

The Importance of Strength Training
As we age, our bodies undergo numerous changes. Muscle mass naturally decreases, a phenomenon known as sarcopenia, which can start as early as our 30s and accelerate after 60. This loss of muscle can lead to decreased strength and endurance, making everyday tasks—like climbing stairs, carrying groceries, or even standing up from a chair—more challenging. Here are some key reasons why strength training is crucial for seniors:

Improved Balance and Stability: Strength training enhances the muscles responsible for maintaining balance, reducing the risk of falls—one of the leading causes of injury in older adults.

Enhanced Joint Health: By strengthening the muscles around your joints, you can alleviate pressure and strain on them, leading to reduced pain and improved function, especially for those with arthritis.

Increased Metabolic Rate: Building muscle increases your resting metabolic rate, meaning you'll burn more calories even while at rest. This can be particularly beneficial for weight management.

Greater Independence: With increased strength and mobility, seniors can maintain their independence longer, allowing them to perform daily activities without assistance.

Mental Well-being: Engaging in strength training releases endorphins, which can improve mood, reduce anxiety, and enhance overall mental health.

Getting Started with Strength Training
Before beginning any new exercise program, it's essential to consult with a healthcare provider, especially if you have existing health conditions or concerns. Once cleared, consider these guidelines for starting your strength training journey:

1. Set Clear Goals
Establish what you want to achieve with strength training. Your goals may include improving overall strength, increasing flexibility, or enhancing specific functional abilities. Setting measurable, attainable goals can help keep you motivated and on track.

2. Choose the Right Environment
Whether you prefer working out at home or in a gym, ensure that your environment is comfortable and equipped with the necessary tools. At home, a sturdy chair, resistance bands, light dumbbells, or even household items like water bottles can serve as effective weights.

3. Warm Up Properly
Before any strength training session, it's vital to warm up your muscles to prevent injury. Spend 5-10 minutes doing light aerobic activity, such as walking or gentle chair exercises, followed by dynamic stretches that target the muscles you plan to work.

Essential Strength Training Exercises for Seniors
Here are some effective strength training exercises specifically designed to enhance functionality in daily life. Each exercise is categorized into upper body, lower body, and core strengthening movements.

Upper Body Exercises
Seated Dumbbell Press

How to do it: Sit on a sturdy chair with a dumbbell in each hand at shoulder height. Slowly press the weights overhead until your arms are fully extended. Lower back to shoulder height.
Benefits: Strengthens the shoulders and arms, which are essential for lifting and reaching activities.
Bicep Curls

How to do it: Sit with a dumbbell in each hand, arms at your sides. Slowly curl the weights toward your shoulders, keeping your elbows close to your body. Lower back down.
Benefits: Enhances arm strength, useful for tasks like carrying bags or lifting items.
Seated Rows with Resistance Bands

How to do it: Sit on the edge of a chair, with a resistance band looped around your feet. Hold the ends and pull them towards you, squeezing your shoulder blades together. Slowly return to the starting position.
Benefits: Improves posture and back strength, crucial for maintaining balance and preventing falls.
Lower Body Exercises
Chair Squats

How to do it: Stand in front of a sturdy chair, feet hip-width apart. Lower your body as if you're going to sit, keeping your weight in your heels, then stand back up.
Benefits: Builds strength in the legs and glutes, aiding in activities like getting up from a seated position.
Seated Leg Lifts

How to do it: While seated, extend one leg out in front of you, holding for a count of five before lowering it back down. Alternate legs.
Benefits: Strengthens the quadriceps and helps improve mobility.
Calf Raises

How to do it: Stand behind a chair, holding onto the back for support. Rise up onto your toes, then slowly lower back down.
Benefits: Strengthens the calves, which is vital for walking and climbing stairs.
Core Exercises
Seated Marches

How to do it: While seated, lift one knee towards your chest, then lower it back down. Alternate legs.
Benefits: Engages the core and improves balance, key for everyday movements.
Torso Twists

How to do it: Sit with your feet firmly on the ground. Hold your arms at chest level and gently twist your torso to the right, then to the left.
Benefits: Enhances flexibility in the spine and strengthens the oblique muscles.
Pelvic Tilts

How to do it: Sit with a straight back. Gently tilt your pelvis forward and back while engaging your core muscles.

Benefits: Strengthens the abdominal muscles and improves lower back support.

Designing Your Strength Training Routine

Frequency and Duration

Aim to perform strength training exercises at least two to three times per week. Each session can last 20-30 minutes, focusing on different muscle groups to allow for recovery. Here's a simple weekly schedule:

Day 1: Upper body and core
Day 2: Lower body
Day 3: Full body (including both upper and lower exercises)

Repetitions and Sets

Start with one to two sets of 8-12 repetitions for each exercise. As you become more comfortable and stronger, gradually increase to three sets or add more resistance.

Safety Tips for Strength Training

Listen to Your Body: If you experience pain (not to be confused with discomfort), stop the exercise immediately. It's essential to distinguish between muscle fatigue and pain that could indicate injury.

Maintain Proper Form: Focus on quality over quantity. Proper form ensures that you're working the intended muscles and reducing the risk of injury.

Rest and Recover: Allow at least one day of rest between strength training sessions targeting the same muscle groups to let your muscles recover and grow stronger.

Strength training is a powerful tool for seniors looking to enhance their everyday functionality. By incorporating these exercises into your routine, you can improve your strength, balance, and overall quality of life. Remember, the journey toward better health and fitness is not a sprint but a marathon. Celebrate small victories along the way, and stay consistent with your training. With dedication and the right approach, you can enjoy an active, independent, and fulfilling life well into your golden years.

Chapter 2: Getting Started Safely and Smartly

Consulting Your Doctor: Exercise Readiness

When it comes to exercise, especially for seniors over 60, understanding your body and its unique needs is crucial. Before embarking on a new fitness journey, consulting your doctor is a vital step. This initial consultation not only ensures your safety but also sets the foundation for a successful exercise regimen tailored to your individual health circumstances. In this chapter, we'll explore why consulting your doctor is essential, what to discuss during your appointment, and how to ensure you are genuinely ready for physical activity.

Why Consult Your Doctor?
Assessing Individual Health Conditions
As we age, our bodies experience a myriad of changes. Chronic conditions such as arthritis, heart disease, diabetes, and osteoporosis become more prevalent. These conditions can significantly impact your ability to exercise safely. A doctor can assess your overall health and evaluate any existing medical conditions that might influence your exercise choices.

Preventing Injuries
Starting a new exercise routine without understanding your limitations can lead to injuries. Seniors are particularly susceptible to strains, sprains, and other injuries due to decreased muscle mass and bone density. Your doctor can help you identify any potential risks and advise on modifications to prevent injuries while still reaping the benefits of exercise.

Understanding Medications
Many seniors take medications that can affect their ability to exercise. Some medications may cause dizziness, fatigue, or muscle weakness. Others can influence your heart rate and blood pressure. Discussing your current medications with your doctor will help you understand how they might affect your exercise routine and whether any adjustments are necessary.

Creating a Baseline
A health check-up can provide a baseline for your fitness journey. Your doctor may recommend tests to evaluate your heart health, lung function, flexibility, and overall physical condition. These benchmarks can guide you in setting realistic and achievable fitness goals and will allow you to measure your progress over time.

What to Discuss During Your Appointment
Your Exercise Goals

Before visiting your doctor, it's helpful to think about what you hope to achieve through exercise. Whether it's losing weight, gaining flexibility, or enhancing overall health, clearly articulating your goals will help your doctor provide tailored advice.

Current Lifestyle and Activity Level
Be prepared to discuss your current lifestyle, including any physical activities you engage in. This includes walking, gardening, swimming, or even household chores. Understanding your current activity level can help your doctor assess how to best incorporate new exercises into your routine.

Medical History
Provide a detailed account of your medical history, including any surgeries, chronic illnesses, or previous injuries. This information is crucial for your doctor to understand your unique health profile and design an appropriate exercise plan.

Specific Concerns
Don't hesitate to voice any concerns you have about starting an exercise program. Whether it's worries about pain, fatigue, or balance issues, open communication is key to addressing these challenges effectively. Your doctor can recommend specific exercises or strategies to overcome these obstacles.

Recommended Types of Exercise
Ask your doctor about the types of exercise that would be most beneficial for you. They may recommend a combination of aerobic exercises, strength training, flexibility workouts, and balance training. Each type of exercise has its benefits and can be tailored to suit your health conditions.

Follow-up Plans
Discuss the importance of follow-up appointments to monitor your progress and adjust your exercise plan as needed. Regular check-ins will allow you to adapt to any changes in your health status or fitness level.

Signs That Indicate You Are Ready to Start Exercising
After consulting with your doctor, they may provide you with guidelines to determine your readiness for exercise. Here are some key indicators:

Stable Health Conditions
If your chronic health conditions are stable and well-managed, this is a positive sign that you may be ready to begin exercising. Your doctor should confirm that your medications and health status allow for increased physical activity.

Ability to Perform Daily Activities
If you can perform daily activities—such as walking, climbing stairs, or doing household chores—without undue fatigue or pain, this indicates a certain level of fitness that can support a new exercise regimen.

Absence of Pain or Discomfort
If you experience no significant pain during daily activities, it suggests that your body is prepared for the challenges of exercise. However, it's important to differentiate between normal discomfort from physical exertion and pain from injury.

Motivation and Mindset
A positive mindset and motivation to engage in physical activity are critical components of readiness. If you're eager to improve your health and willing to commit to an exercise routine, you're likely in a good place to start.

Support System
Having a support system, whether it's friends, family, or exercise groups, can enhance your readiness. Social support can provide encouragement and motivation, making it easier to stick to your exercise goals.

Tailoring Your Exercise Program
Once you have your doctor's approval, the next step is to tailor your exercise program to fit your unique needs. Here are some key components to consider:

Start Slowly
Begin with low-impact exercises that are easy on the joints, such as walking, swimming, or chair yoga. Gradually increase the intensity and duration of your workouts as your strength and stamina improve.

Incorporate Variety
Mix different types of exercises to keep your routine interesting and comprehensive. Aim to include aerobic, strength, flexibility, and balance exercises in your weekly routine.

Listen to Your Body
Pay attention to how your body responds to exercise. If you experience pain, dizziness, or any other concerning symptoms, stop exercising and consult your doctor.

Stay Consistent

Consistency is key to reaping the benefits of exercise. Aim to incorporate physical activity into your daily routine, setting aside time for workouts and making them a priority.

Reassess Regularly
Regularly reassess your exercise plan with your doctor or fitness expert. Adjust your routine based on your progress, changes in your health, and any new goals you set.

Consulting your doctor before starting a new exercise program is not just a precaution—it's a necessary step to ensure your safety and success. By taking the time to assess your health, discuss your goals, and tailor your routine, you're setting yourself up for a rewarding journey toward improved fitness, flexibility, and overall well-being. Remember, at any age, it's never too late to begin a healthier, more active lifestyle. Embrace this opportunity, listen to your body, and enjoy the process of becoming your best self!

Understanding Your Body's Needs: Flexibility vs. Strength

As we age, our bodies undergo a variety of changes that affect our physical capabilities, including flexibility and strength. Understanding these needs is crucial for developing an effective exercise routine tailored to seniors over 60. This chapter will explore the importance of flexibility and strength, how they differ, and how to create a balanced fitness regimen that addresses both areas.

The Importance of Flexibility
Flexibility refers to the ability of our joints and muscles to move through their full range of motion. As we age, connective tissues lose elasticity, and our muscles may shorten, leading to stiffness. This can impact our ability to perform daily activities, from reaching for something on a high shelf to bending down to tie our shoes.

Why Flexibility Matters:

Injury Prevention: Adequate flexibility can reduce the risk of injuries. Stiff muscles are more prone to strains and sprains. By incorporating stretching and flexibility exercises into your routine, you help your muscles and joints withstand daily stressors, thus minimizing the chance of injury.

Enhanced Performance: Flexibility allows for improved performance in physical activities. Whether you're gardening, walking, or participating in sports, better flexibility can enhance your movement efficiency and make these tasks feel easier.

Improved Posture: As we age, maintaining good posture becomes increasingly important. Tight muscles can lead to postural imbalances, which can cause discomfort and pain. Regular stretching can counteract this, leading to better alignment of the body.

Reduced Pain and Discomfort: Stiffness can often lead to pain, particularly in the back, hips, and shoulders. Stretching helps relieve tension and can reduce discomfort, contributing to an overall sense of well-being.

The Importance of Strength
Strength, on the other hand, refers to the muscle's ability to exert force. As we age, we naturally lose muscle mass and strength, a condition known as sarcopenia. This can affect mobility, balance, and overall functional ability, making it essential to incorporate strength training into your exercise routine.

Why Strength Matters:

Maintaining Independence: Strength training is crucial for maintaining the ability to perform daily activities independently. Tasks such as lifting groceries, climbing stairs, or even getting up from a chair require a certain level of strength. Strength training helps ensure you can continue to perform these activities without assistance.

Improved Bone Density: Engaging in strength training can help prevent osteoporosis by increasing bone density. This is especially important for women over 60, who are at a higher risk for osteoporosis and fractures.

Better Balance and Stability: Strength training not only improves muscle mass but also enhances coordination and balance. This can significantly reduce the risk of falls, which are a leading cause of injury among seniors.

Boosted Metabolism: Muscle tissue burns more calories than fat tissue, even at rest. Therefore, maintaining muscle mass through strength training can help keep your metabolism active, making weight management easier as you age.

Flexibility vs. Strength: Finding the Right Balance

Both flexibility and strength are vital components of a well-rounded fitness program, especially for seniors. However, the right balance will depend on individual needs, goals, and current fitness levels.

Assessing Your Current Fitness Level: Before embarking on any exercise program, it's crucial to assess your current flexibility and strength levels. This can be done through simple tests, such as the sit-and-reach test for flexibility or the chair stand test for strength. Understanding your baseline will help tailor a program that addresses your specific needs.

Listening to Your Body: It's essential to pay attention to how your body feels during exercises. If you experience pain, it may be a sign that you're pushing too hard. Conversely, if you feel capable of handling more, it may be time to progress your routine. Always prioritize safety and avoid comparing yourself to others.

Incorporating Both Components: A balanced routine should include both strength training and flexibility exercises. This might look like alternating days between strength training and stretching or combining both in a single workout session. For instance, you can perform a set of strength exercises followed by a series of stretches to enhance recovery and maintain flexibility.

Choosing the Right Exercises: The best exercises for you will depend on your current fitness level and any physical limitations.

For Flexibility: Consider gentle yoga or chair yoga poses, dynamic stretching, or guided stretching routines specifically designed for seniors. Poses like the seated forward bend, gentle twists, and shoulder stretches are excellent starting points.

For Strength: Focus on body-weight exercises, resistance bands, or light weights. Exercises such as seated leg lifts, chair squats, and bicep curls are accessible yet effective for building strength.

Set Realistic Goals: It's essential to set achievable goals based on your assessments. This might include improving flexibility by a certain number of inches in a month or being able to perform a specific number of chair squats without assistance.

Consistency is Key: Establish a regular workout schedule that allows you to work on both flexibility and strength. Aim for at least two to three days of strength training per week, along with flexibility exercises on most days.

Understanding your body's needs for flexibility and strength is essential as you age. By prioritizing both components in your fitness routine, you can enhance your overall health, improve your quality of life, and maintain your independence. Remember, it's not about achieving perfection but rather about making consistent, gradual progress toward a healthier you.

The journey to improved flexibility and strength is a personal one, and it's never too late to start. With patience, dedication, and the right mindset, you can cultivate a fitness routine that empowers you and helps you thrive well into your golden years.

Recommended Next Steps:
Consult with a Fitness Professional: Consider working with a certified trainer who specializes in senior fitness to help you develop a personalized plan.

Join a Class: Participating in a chair yoga or strength training class can provide the guidance and support you need, as well as a sense of community.

Stay Informed: Continuously educate yourself about best practices for senior fitness and adapt your routine as your body changes.

By embracing both flexibility and strength, you are not just investing in your physical health; you are enhancing your ability to enjoy life fully and actively.

Setting Realistic Fitness Goals: Weight Loss and Beyond

Setting fitness goals can be both exciting and daunting, especially for seniors over 60. Whether you're just starting your fitness journey or looking to enhance your current routine, understanding how to set realistic and achievable goals is crucial. We'll explore the significance of goal setting, how to tailor these goals to your unique situation, and practical strategies to keep you motivated and on track.

The Importance of Setting Goals
Setting fitness goals serves several important purposes:

Direction and Purpose: Goals provide a clear focus for your exercise efforts. Instead of going through the motions, you'll have a destination to work towards.

Motivation: When you have specific goals, you're more likely to stay motivated. Each milestone achieved can boost your confidence and encourage you to continue.

Accountability: Sharing your goals with friends, family, or a fitness community can create a support system that holds you accountable.

Measure Progress: Goals allow you to track your progress over time, which can be incredibly rewarding. Seeing tangible results, whether in weight loss, increased flexibility, or improved strength, reinforces your commitment.

Understanding Your Starting Point
Before setting your goals, it's essential to understand where you're starting from. Consider the following:

Assess Your Current Fitness Level
Physical Activity Assessment: Take note of how active you currently are. Are you engaging in regular physical activity, or are you starting from a sedentary lifestyle? Assess your flexibility, strength, and endurance through simple movements like standing up from a chair, reaching for your toes, or walking around your home.

Health Considerations: Consult with a healthcare professional to understand any limitations you may have due to existing health conditions. This step is particularly important for seniors, as certain exercises may need to be modified for safety.

Emotional Readiness: Recognize your mental and emotional readiness for a fitness journey. Are you feeling motivated to make changes? Understanding your mindset can help you choose goals that align with your current emotional state.

Reflect on Your Personal Motivations
Identifying why you want to achieve your fitness goals is vital. For instance, do you want to lose weight for health reasons, to have more energy, or to participate in activities with family and friends? Reflecting on your motivations will help you set goals that resonate with you personally.

Setting SMART Goals
One effective framework for goal setting is the SMART criteria, which stands for Specific, Measurable, Achievable, Relevant, and Time-bound. Let's break down each component:

Specific: Define your goals clearly. Instead of saying, "I want to lose weight," try "I want to lose 10 pounds." Specificity gives you a clear target.

Measurable: Choose goals that you can measure easily. This might include tracking the number of exercises completed, pounds lost, or distances walked.

Achievable: Set goals that are realistic based on your current fitness level and lifestyle. Aiming to lose 30 pounds in a month might not be feasible, but losing 1-2 pounds a week is much more attainable.

Relevant: Ensure your goals align with your personal motivations and overall health objectives. If your primary concern is joint health, consider incorporating flexibility and strength training into your goals.

Time-bound: Set a timeframe for your goals. For example, "I want to lose 10 pounds in three months." A timeline adds urgency and encourages consistent effort.

Example of a SMART Goal
Instead of setting a vague goal like "I want to get fit," a SMART goal might look like this:
"I want to lose 10 pounds in 12 weeks by exercising three times a week and eating a balanced diet focused on fruits and vegetables."

Creating a Balanced Approach to Fitness Goals
While weight loss is often a primary focus, it's crucial to create a balanced approach that considers other aspects of health and fitness. Here are some additional goals to consider:

Increase Flexibility: Aim to incorporate stretching or yoga into your routine. A goal might be to perform a specific stretch for 10 minutes every day or to participate in a weekly chair yoga class.

Build Strength: Set a goal to incorporate strength training exercises into your routine, such as chair squats or resistance band exercises. For instance, "I will complete a 20-minute strength training session twice a week."

Enhance Endurance: Focus on cardiovascular health by setting goals related to walking or other aerobic activities. For example, "I want to walk for 30 minutes, five times a week."

Improve Balance and Coordination: Balance exercises can significantly reduce the risk of falls. Consider setting a goal to practice balance exercises, such as standing on one leg, for five minutes each day.

Nutrition Goals: Pairing fitness goals with nutrition can enhance your results. Aim for goals like "I will eat at least two servings of vegetables with each meal" or "I will drink eight glasses of water a day."

Tracking Your Progress

To maintain motivation, tracking your progress is essential. Here are some strategies to help you do this effectively:

Keep a Journal: Document your workouts, meals, and any changes in your weight or flexibility. Reflect on what is working and what needs adjustment.

Use Technology: Fitness apps and wearable devices can help you monitor your activity levels, track your weight loss, and log your workouts. They can provide reminders and encouragement along the way.

Celebrate Small Wins: Recognize and celebrate your achievements, no matter how small. Every step forward counts, whether it's fitting into a favorite pair of pants or completing a challenging exercise.

Overcoming Challenges and Staying Motivated
As you pursue your fitness goals, you may encounter challenges. Here are some strategies to stay motivated:

Be Flexible: Life can be unpredictable. If you miss a workout or have an off day, don't be too hard on yourself. Adjust your goals and get back on track without guilt.

Find Support: Engage friends, family, or local fitness groups. Having a support system can provide encouragement, accountability, and companionship during your fitness journey.

Stay Positive: Focus on the positives of your journey, such as increased energy, improved mood, or enhanced mobility. A positive mindset can significantly impact your commitment to your goals.

Mix It Up: Keep your routine fresh and exciting by trying new exercises or activities. This can prevent boredom and keep you engaged in your fitness journey.

Visualize Success: Spend a few moments each day visualizing yourself achieving your goals. Imagine the feelings of accomplishment and satisfaction that come with your success.

Setting realistic fitness goals is a powerful tool for achieving weight loss and enhancing your overall health and well-being as a senior. By understanding your starting point, employing the SMART framework, and adopting a balanced approach, you can create goals that motivate and inspire you.

Remember, it's not just about the destination but also the journey. Celebrate each step you take towards your goals and embrace the positive changes that come with an active lifestyle. By making fitness a priority, you can improve your quality of life, gain strength, and enjoy the many benefits of staying active after 60.

Creating a Comfortable Space at Home for Exercise and What You'll Need

When it comes to staying active, especially for seniors over 60, having a designated exercise space at home can make all the difference. A comfortable, inviting environment not only encourages regular activity but also promotes a sense of safety and well-being. Whether you're starting a chair yoga routine, engaging in strength training, or simply stretching, setting up your space thoughtfully can enhance your experience and boost your motivation. Let's explore how to create that ideal exercise space.

1. Choosing the Right Location
Finding the Perfect Spot
Start by identifying a location in your home that is spacious enough to accommodate your exercises. This could be a corner of your living room, a spare room, or even a sunlit area in the backyard. Look for a spot that is:

Well-Lit: Natural light can uplift your mood and enhance focus. If possible, choose a location with windows to let in sunlight. If not, consider adding soft artificial lighting that is easy on the eyes.

Quiet and Free from Distractions: Choose an area away from the hustle and bustle of daily life. Reducing noise and interruptions will help you concentrate on your movements and breathing.

Accessible: Make sure the space is easy to access. You don't want to navigate stairs or awkward corners each time you want to exercise.

2. Safety First: Ensuring a Secure Environment
Clear the Space
Before you start arranging your area, ensure it is free from clutter. Remove any items that could pose a tripping hazard, such as:

Rugs or carpets that might slip
Cables and wires
Furniture with sharp edges
Small decor items that can easily be knocked over
Flooring Matters
The type of flooring can significantly impact your comfort. If you have hard surfaces like tile or hardwood, consider using a yoga mat or exercise mat for added cushioning. This will help absorb

impact during exercises and provide stability, especially during seated movements. If possible, choose a space with non-slip flooring to enhance safety further.

3. Essential Equipment for Your Home Workout
Invest in Basic Equipment
While your body is the primary tool for many exercises, having a few essential pieces of equipment can enrich your routine. Here's a list of items to consider:

Sturdy Chair: A solid, comfortable chair is crucial for chair yoga and strength exercises. Ensure it is stable and at a height that allows your feet to rest flat on the floor when seated.

Weights: Light dumbbells (1-5 pounds) or resistance bands can be easily stored and are effective for strength training. Start with lighter weights and gradually increase as you build strength.

Yoga Mat: A non-slip yoga mat is essential if you plan on doing floor exercises or stretches. It provides comfort and helps you maintain balance during your workouts.

Water Bottle: Hydration is vital, especially during physical activity. Keep a water bottle nearby to ensure you stay refreshed.

Exercise Journal: Documenting your progress can help maintain motivation. Consider keeping a notebook or planner in your exercise area to track your workouts and feelings.

4. Personalizing Your Space
Adding Comfort and Inspiration
Creating an inviting atmosphere can greatly enhance your workout experience. Consider these personalization tips:

Incorporate Plants: Indoor plants can purify the air and add a touch of nature to your workout space. Consider low-maintenance options like succulents or peace lilies.

Art and Inspiration: Hang motivational quotes or artwork that inspires you. This could be photos of loved ones, affirmations about health, or images that evoke peace and motivation.

Ambient Music: Music can elevate your mood and enhance your workout experience. Consider setting up a small speaker or using a portable device to play calming music or guided workouts.

Comfortable Clothing: Ensure you have comfortable, breathable clothing designated for your workout sessions. This will help you feel more at ease and focused on your exercises.

5. Establishing a Routine
Creating a Consistent Schedule

Once your space is set up, it's time to establish a routine. Consistency is key to developing a lasting exercise habit. Here's how to integrate your new space into your daily life:

Set Specific Times: Designate specific times for your workouts. Whether it's morning stretches or evening chair yoga, having a routine helps your body adapt to regular movement.

Start Small: If you're new to exercising or have had a long break, begin with short sessions (10-15 minutes) and gradually increase the duration. This prevents burnout and discouragement.

Use Visual Reminders: Place reminders in your exercise area, such as post-it notes with your workout schedule or motivational quotes. These can serve as prompts to encourage you to stick with your routine.

6. Inviting Others to Join
Making It a Social Activity

Exercising with others can make the experience more enjoyable and motivating. If you feel comfortable, invite friends or family to join you in your workout space. Here are some ideas for social exercise:

Group Chair Yoga Sessions: Set a time each week for a chair yoga class with friends. This can be done in person or virtually, allowing you to connect with loved ones no matter the distance.

Buddy System for Strength Training: Pair up with a friend for strength training. You can encourage one another and share tips, making workouts feel less daunting and more fun.

7. Listening to Your Body
Prioritizing Your Comfort and Health

As you create this space, remember that listening to your body is essential. Here are a few tips:

Modify When Necessary: If a certain exercise feels uncomfortable or painful, don't hesitate to modify it or skip it altogether. It's crucial to find movements that work for your body.

Rest and Recovery: Allow your body adequate time to rest. Include days dedicated to relaxation and recovery in your routine, and be sure to engage in gentle stretching or meditation to maintain flexibility and mental clarity.

Creating a comfortable and functional exercise space at home is an investment in your health and well-being. By selecting the right location, ensuring safety, incorporating essential equipment, and personalizing your environment, you set the stage for a successful and enjoyable workout routine. Embrace the journey, listen to your body, and remember that every small effort contributes to your overall wellness. The most important thing is to keep moving, enjoying the process, and celebrating your progress—no matter how small.

Chapter 3: Chair Yoga for Beginners

What is Chair Yoga?

Chair yoga is a gentle form of yoga that is practiced while seated in a chair or while using a chair for support during standing poses. It is designed to provide the benefits of traditional yoga to individuals who may have limited mobility, balance issues, or other physical challenges that make standard yoga practices difficult. This makes chair yoga particularly popular among seniors, those recovering from injuries, and anyone seeking a more accessible way to engage in physical activity and mindfulness.

The Origins of Chair Yoga
The concept of chair yoga emerged as a response to the growing need for inclusive fitness programs that accommodate individuals with varying levels of ability. As yoga gained popularity in the Western world, instructors began to recognize that many people were unable to participate in traditional yoga classes due to physical limitations. This led to the development of chair yoga, which maintains the fundamental principles of yoga—such as breath control, flexibility, strength, and mindfulness—while adapting the poses and sequences to make them accessible.

The Benefits of Chair Yoga
Improved Flexibility and Range of Motion
One of the primary benefits of chair yoga is its ability to enhance flexibility. The gentle stretching and movement encouraged by chair yoga can help improve the range of motion in joints, which is particularly important for seniors or individuals with conditions like arthritis. By incorporating various seated and supported stretches, chair yoga promotes the elongation of muscles and increases joint flexibility.

Increased Strength and Stability
Chair yoga not only focuses on stretching but also incorporates strength-building exercises. Many poses engage core muscles and support overall body strength, which can help improve balance and stability. This is crucial for preventing falls, a common concern for older adults. Exercises such as seated leg lifts and arm raises target different muscle groups and contribute to functional strength, making everyday activities easier.

Enhanced Circulation

Gentle movements and stretches promote better blood circulation throughout the body. Improved circulation can help alleviate discomfort and stiffness, increase energy levels, and support overall cardiovascular health. This is especially beneficial for individuals who may have sedentary lifestyles or are unable to engage in more vigorous forms of exercise.

Stress Reduction and Mental Clarity

Chair yoga is not just about physical movement; it also emphasizes breath control and mindfulness. Focusing on the breath and being present in the moment can significantly reduce stress and anxiety levels. Regular practice fosters a sense of calm and promotes mental clarity, making it an excellent tool for enhancing emotional well-being.

Adaptability and Accessibility

One of the greatest strengths of chair yoga is its adaptability. Almost anyone can practice chair yoga, regardless of their fitness level or physical limitations. Whether seated or using a chair for support, individuals can modify poses to suit their comfort and ability. This inclusivity allows people to experience the benefits of yoga without the fear of injury or strain.

Key Principles of Chair Yoga

Breath Awareness

Breath is a central component of yoga practice. In chair yoga, practitioners are encouraged to focus on their breath, using deep, intentional inhalations and exhalations to connect movement with breath. This not only enhances the physical practice but also encourages relaxation and mindfulness.

Mindfulness and Presence

Chair yoga promotes mindfulness by encouraging participants to be fully present in their bodies and movements. This practice of awareness helps individuals connect their mind and body, leading to a deeper understanding of their physical capabilities and limitations.

Gentle Movement

The movements in chair yoga are slow, controlled, and gentle, making them suitable for individuals of all fitness levels. Practitioners are encouraged to listen to their bodies and avoid pushing themselves beyond their comfort zones.

Modifications and Variations

In chair yoga, modifications are encouraged to accommodate individual needs. For instance, if a participant cannot perform a standing pose, they may remain seated or use the chair for balance. This principle empowers practitioners to take charge of their practice and ensure it suits their unique abilities.

Common Chair Yoga Poses

Here are some commonly practiced chair yoga poses that illustrate the diversity and accessibility of this form of yoga:

Seated Mountain Pose (Tadasana)

Sit up tall with your feet flat on the ground, hip-width apart.
Lengthen your spine, relax your shoulders, and rest your hands on your thighs.
Take several deep breaths, focusing on grounding your body and lifting through the crown of your head.

Seated Forward Bend (Paschimottanasana)

While seated, extend your legs in front of you with your feet flexed.
Inhale as you reach your arms overhead, and exhale as you hinge at the hips to fold forward, reaching for your feet or shins.
Hold the stretch for a few breaths, feeling the gentle elongation in your spine and hamstrings.

Chair Twist (Ardha Matsyendrasana)

Sit tall in your chair and place your right hand on the back of the chair.
Inhale as you lengthen your spine, and exhale as you gently twist to the right, using your hand for support.
Hold for several breaths, then return to center and repeat on the left side.

Seated Cat-Cow Stretch

Sit at the edge of your chair with your feet flat on the floor.
Inhale as you arch your back and lift your chest (Cow), and exhale as you round your spine and tuck your chin (Cat).
Continue this flow for several breaths, synchronizing your movements with your breath.

Seated Leg Lifts

While seated, extend one leg out in front of you, keeping it straight.
Hold for a few breaths, then lower it back down.
Repeat on the other side to strengthen your legs and improve balance.

Integrating Chair Yoga into Daily Life

Chair yoga can be easily integrated into daily routines, making it a practical choice for individuals seeking to maintain or improve their physical health. Here are some tips for incorporating chair yoga into your life:

Set a Regular Schedule
Consistency is key to experiencing the benefits of chair yoga. Aim to practice for 10-20 minutes daily or a few times a week, depending on your schedule and comfort level.

Create a Comfortable Space
Designate a quiet, comfortable space in your home for practice. Ensure you have a sturdy chair with no arms and a clear area to move. You might also want to have a yoga mat or cushion nearby for added comfort.

Join a Class
Look for local classes or online sessions focused on chair yoga. Participating in a group can enhance motivation and provide the opportunity to learn from experienced instructors.

Practice Mindfulness Throughout the Day
Incorporate breath awareness and mindfulness into your daily activities. Whether you're cooking, walking, or sitting, take moments to connect with your breath and appreciate the present.

Encourage Others
Chair yoga can be a social activity. Invite friends or family to join you in a session. Practicing together can enhance motivation and create a supportive environment.

Chair yoga offers a remarkable way to experience the benefits of yoga, regardless of physical limitations. By focusing on gentle movement, breath awareness, and mindfulness, individuals can enhance their flexibility, strength, and overall well-being. This accessible practice empowers seniors and those with mobility challenges to engage in physical activity, cultivate a sense of community, and improve their quality of life. As you embark on your chair yoga journey, remember that every breath and every movement is a step toward greater health and happiness. Whether you're new to yoga or returning after a break, chair yoga welcomes you with open arms—right from your seat.

Breathing and Mindfulness Techniques

As we age, maintaining both physical and mental well-being becomes increasingly important. One of the most powerful yet often overlooked tools at our disposal is our breath. Incorporating breathing exercises and mindfulness techniques into your daily routine can significantly enhance your overall health, especially for seniors. These practices not only improve physical health but also foster mental clarity and emotional stability. This section we will delve into the art of breathing and mindfulness, providing you with a comprehensive guide to understanding and implementing these techniques in your life.

Understanding the Breath

Breathing is an automatic process, but how often do we truly pay attention to it? Proper breathing techniques can help alleviate stress, enhance relaxation, and even improve physical performance. The breath serves as a bridge between the body and mind, allowing us to influence our physiological state through mindful practice.

The Anatomy of Breathing

To appreciate the power of our breath, it's essential to understand the mechanics behind it. Breathing involves several key components:

Diaphragm: This dome-shaped muscle located beneath the lungs plays a crucial role in respiration. When you inhale, the diaphragm contracts, allowing the lungs to expand and fill with air. A proper diaphragmatic breath engages the entire body.

Intercostal Muscles: These muscles are located between the ribs and assist in expanding and contracting the rib cage. Engaging these muscles can enhance lung capacity and improve oxygen intake.

Nasal Passages: Breathing through the nose filters, warms, and humidifies the air, making it more suitable for the lungs. It also helps regulate the breath's depth and rhythm.

The Benefits of Mindful Breathing

Mindful breathing can provide numerous benefits:

Stress Reduction: Focusing on your breath activates the parasympathetic nervous system, which promotes relaxation and reduces the production of stress hormones like cortisol.

Improved Mental Clarity: Concentrating on your breath helps clear mental clutter, enhancing focus and cognitive function.

Emotional Regulation: By cultivating awareness of your breath, you can gain better control over your emotions, leading to improved mood and emotional stability.

Enhanced Physical Health: Mindful breathing techniques can improve lung function, enhance circulation, and promote better sleep.

Breathing Techniques

Now that we understand the importance of breath, let's explore some effective breathing techniques tailored for seniors. These exercises are designed to be gentle, accessible, and beneficial for overall health.

Diaphragmatic Breathing (Belly Breathing)

This technique promotes full oxygen exchange and engages the diaphragm, providing a calming effect.

How to Do It:
Find a comfortable position—either sitting or lying down.
Place one hand on your chest and the other on your belly.
Inhale deeply through your nose, allowing your belly to rise while keeping your chest relatively still.
Exhale slowly through your mouth, feeling your belly fall.
Repeat for 5-10 minutes, focusing on the rise and fall of your belly.
4-7-8 Breathing Technique

This method helps induce a state of relaxation and is particularly effective before sleep.

How to Do It:
Sit or lie down in a comfortable position.
Close your eyes and take a deep breath in through your nose for 4 counts.
Hold your breath for 7 counts.
Exhale slowly through your mouth for 8 counts, making a whooshing sound.
Repeat the cycle for 4-8 rounds.
Box Breathing

Also known as square breathing, this technique helps with focus and stress reduction.

How to Do It:
Sit comfortably with your back straight.
Inhale through your nose for a count of 4.
Hold your breath for a count of 4.
Exhale through your mouth for a count of 4.

Hold your breath again for a count of 4.
Repeat the cycle for several minutes.

Alternate Nostril Breathing (Nadi Shodhana)

This technique balances the body's energies and calms the mind.

How to Do It:
Sit comfortably with your spine straight.
Use your right thumb to close your right nostril.
Inhale deeply through your left nostril.
Close your left nostril with your right ring finger and release your right nostril.
Exhale through your right nostril.
Inhale through the right nostril, close it, and exhale through the left nostril.
Continue alternating for several minutes.

Incorporating Mindfulness

In addition to breathing exercises, cultivating mindfulness is essential for enhancing mental well-being. Mindfulness involves being present in the moment without judgment. It encourages a deeper awareness of your thoughts, feelings, and bodily sensations, fostering a sense of calm and clarity.

Mindfulness Meditation

This practice helps develop a more profound awareness of the present moment.

How to Do It:
Find a quiet place where you won't be disturbed.
Sit comfortably with your back straight and hands resting on your knees.
Close your eyes and take a few deep breaths to center yourself.
Focus your attention on your breath—notice the sensations of inhaling and exhaling.
When your mind wanders (which it will), gently guide your focus back to your breath.
Start with 5 minutes and gradually increase the duration as you become more comfortable.

Mindful Movement

Integrating mindfulness into your daily activities can be incredibly beneficial. Whether you are walking, eating, or even exercising, focus on the sensations, sounds, and smells associated with the activity.

How to Practice:

During a walk, pay attention to the feeling of your feet on the ground, the air on your skin, and the sounds around you.

While eating, savor each bite, noting the flavors and textures without distractions like TV or smartphones.

Combining Breathing and Mindfulness

The true power of breathing and mindfulness techniques comes when they are combined. By integrating these practices into your daily routine, you can create a holistic approach to well-being. Here's how to combine them effectively:

Mindful Breathing Practice
Set aside a few minutes each day to practice mindful breathing. As you focus on your breath, notice the thoughts that arise without judgment. Acknowledge them and gently bring your focus back to your breath.

Create a Routine
Incorporate breathing and mindfulness practices into your existing routines. For example, practice diaphragmatic breathing while you prepare meals or use box breathing during moments of stress throughout the day.

Set Intentions
Before starting any breathing or mindfulness practice, take a moment to set an intention. This could be a simple phrase like "I am calm" or "I am present." Revisit this intention throughout your practice to deepen your focus.

Journaling
After each practice session, take a few minutes to journal your thoughts and feelings. Reflect on how the practice made you feel and any insights gained. This will help reinforce the benefits of mindfulness and breathing techniques.

Breathing and mindfulness techniques are powerful tools for enhancing both physical and mental well-being, especially for seniors. By embracing these practices, you can foster a deeper connection to your body and mind, leading to improved health, reduced stress, and greater emotional resilience. Start incorporating these techniques into your daily routine today, and experience the transformative effects they can have on your life. Remember, it's never too late to cultivate mindfulness and harness the power of your breath. Your journey towards a healthier, more balanced life begins with just a few breaths.

Simple Chair Yoga Poses for Flexibility

Chair yoga is an excellent way for seniors and individuals of all ages to enhance flexibility, strength, and overall well-being. It provides a safe, supportive environment for those who may have difficulty performing traditional yoga poses on the floor. Whether you're a beginner or someone looking to maintain your routine, these simple chair yoga poses can help you improve flexibility, reduce stress, and enhance your overall quality of life.

The Benefits of Chair Yoga
Before diving into the poses, it's essential to understand the benefits of chair yoga. Unlike traditional yoga, chair yoga allows you to perform exercises while seated, making it accessible for those with limited mobility or balance issues. Here are some key benefits:

Improved Flexibility: Regular practice of chair yoga can help stretch and lengthen muscles, increasing your overall flexibility and range of motion.

Enhanced Strength: Many poses involve using your body weight to build strength, particularly in the core and lower body.

Stress Reduction: The combination of gentle movements, deep breathing, and mindfulness promotes relaxation and helps alleviate anxiety.

Increased Balance and Stability: Chair yoga helps improve your balance, reducing the risk of falls, which is especially important for seniors.

Enhanced Circulation: Gentle movements promote blood flow, which can help reduce stiffness and increase energy levels.

Preparing for Chair Yoga
Before starting your chair yoga practice, ensure you have a sturdy chair without arms that can support your movements. A chair with a cushion can also provide additional comfort. Here's how to set up your space:

Choose the Right Chair: A kitchen or dining chair without arms is ideal. Make sure it is stable and at a height that allows your feet to rest flat on the floor.

Create a Comfortable Environment: Find a quiet space where you won't be disturbed. You may want to play soft music or use calming scents like lavender to enhance relaxation.

Dress Comfortably: Wear loose-fitting clothing that allows for free movement. Avoid tight or restrictive clothing that may hinder your stretches.

Use a Yoga Mat or Non-Slip Surface: If you're concerned about stability, consider placing a yoga mat or a non-slip surface under your chair to prevent any sliding.

Hydrate: Drink water before and after your session to stay hydrated.

Simple Chair Yoga Poses
Now, let's explore some simple chair yoga poses that can help enhance flexibility. Each pose is designed to be gentle and can be modified according to your comfort level.

1. Seated Mountain Pose (Tadasana)
Benefits: This pose helps improve posture, promotes stability, and enhances focus.

How to Perform:

Sit up straight in your chair, with your feet flat on the floor, hip-width apart.
Place your hands on your thighs, palms facing down.
Take a deep breath in, raising your arms overhead, with palms facing each other.
Hold the pose for a few breaths, focusing on lengthening your spine and relaxing your shoulders.
Exhale slowly as you lower your arms back to your thighs.
Duration: Hold for 5-10 breaths.

2. Seated Forward Bend (Paschimottanasana)
Benefits: This pose stretches the back, hamstrings, and calves, promoting overall flexibility.

How to Perform:

Sit tall with your feet flat on the floor, shoulder-width apart.
Inhale, lengthening your spine and reaching your arms overhead.
As you exhale, hinge at the hips and lean forward, reaching for your feet or shins.
Keep your back straight, and don't force the stretch. Go only as far as comfortable.
Allow your head to hang gently towards your knees.
Duration: Hold for 5-10 breaths, feeling the stretch in your back and legs.

3. Seated Cat-Cow Stretch
Benefits: This dynamic pose promotes flexibility in the spine and helps alleviate tension in the back.

How to Perform:

Sit on the edge of your chair with your feet flat on the ground.
Inhale, arching your back and lifting your chest (Cow Pose).
Exhale, rounding your spine and tucking your chin towards your chest (Cat Pose).
Continue this movement, flowing between the two positions with each breath.
Duration: Perform for 5-8 cycles.

4. Seated Side Stretch
Benefits: This pose increases flexibility in the side body and improves spinal mobility.

How to Perform:

Sit tall with your feet flat on the floor.
Inhale, raising your right arm overhead, reaching towards the ceiling.
Exhale, leaning gently to the left, feeling a stretch along your right side.
Hold the stretch for a few breaths, focusing on your breath.
Inhale to come back to center and switch sides, repeating the stretch on the right.
Duration: Hold each side for 5 breaths.

5. Seated Leg Extension
Benefits: This pose strengthens the quadriceps and improves flexibility in the hamstrings.

How to Perform:

Sit tall in your chair, feet flat on the floor.
Inhale, extending your right leg out in front of you until it is parallel to the ground.
Flex your foot, pressing through the heel.
Hold for a few breaths, then lower your leg back down.
Repeat on the left side.
Duration: Hold each leg for 5 breaths.

6. Seated Spinal Twist
Benefits: This pose increases spinal flexibility and aids digestion.

How to Perform:

Sit tall with your feet flat on the floor.
Inhale, lengthening your spine.

Exhale, twisting your torso to the right, placing your left hand on your right knee and your right hand on the back of the chair.
Hold for a few breaths, then return to center and repeat on the left side.
Duration: Hold each side for 5 breaths.

7. Seated Ankle Circles
Benefits: This pose promotes ankle flexibility and helps improve circulation in the legs.

How to Perform:

Sit with your feet flat on the floor.
Extend your right leg out slightly and lift your foot off the ground.
Move your foot in a circular motion, making ten circles clockwise and then counterclockwise.
Lower your leg and repeat on the left side.
Duration: Perform 10 circles each direction on both legs.

8. Seated Wrist and Finger Stretch
Benefits: This pose helps alleviate tension in the wrists and fingers, promoting flexibility.

How to Perform:

Sit tall with your feet flat on the ground.
Extend your right arm in front of you, palm facing up.
With your left hand, gently pull back on your fingers, feeling a stretch in your wrist and forearm.
Hold for a few breaths, then switch to the left side.
Duration: Hold each side for 5 breaths.

Cool Down: Relaxation and Breathing
After completing your chair yoga poses, it's essential to cool down and bring your body back to a state of rest:

Seated Relaxation: Sit comfortably with your feet flat on the floor and your hands resting in your lap. Close your eyes and take several deep breaths. Focus on inhaling deeply through your nose and exhaling slowly through your mouth.

Visualization: Picture a peaceful scene, such as a beach or a serene forest. Spend a few moments immersing yourself in this calming image as you continue to breathe deeply.

Gratitude Reflection: Take a moment to reflect on what you are grateful for today. Acknowledge the positive aspects of your life, which can enhance your overall sense of well-being.

Incorporating Chair Yoga into Your Routine
To fully reap the benefits of chair yoga, consider incorporating these poses into your daily routine. Aim to practice chair yoga 3-5 times a week, even if it's for just 10-15 minutes each session. You can gradually increase the duration as you become more comfortable with the poses.

Tips for Success
Listen to Your Body: Always pay attention to how your body feels. If a pose causes discomfort, modify it or skip it altogether.
Practice Mindfulness: Focus on your breath and the sensations in your body. Mindfulness enhances the benefits of yoga and promotes relaxation.
Stay Consistent: Consistency is key to seeing progress. Set a regular schedule for your practice to help you stay motivated.
Use Props If Needed: If you find certain poses challenging, don't hesitate to use props like straps or blankets to assist you.

Chair yoga is a fantastic way to enhance flexibility, reduce stress, and improve overall health for seniors and anyone seeking a gentle yet effective form of exercise. With the simple chair yoga poses outlined above, you can easily integrate this practice into your daily routine, helping you feel more balanced, stronger, and more flexible. Remember to listen to your body and enjoy the process of movement and mindfulness as you embark on your chair yoga journey. Embrace each moment, and celebrate the positive changes that come with consistent practice.

Seated Cat-Cow Stretch

The Seated Cat-Cow Stretch is a gentle yet effective exercise that combines movement with mindful breathing, making it an ideal choice for seniors looking to enhance flexibility, relieve tension, and promote spinal health. This stretch can be performed in the comfort of your home, using a sturdy chair for support. It targets the spine, neck, and shoulders, fostering better posture and increased range of motion, which can be particularly beneficial as we age.

Benefits of the Seated Cat-Cow Stretch
Improves Spinal Flexibility: The Cat-Cow Stretch encourages the natural flexion and extension of the spine, enhancing overall spinal mobility.

Relieves Tension: This movement helps alleviate tightness in the back and neck, common areas of discomfort for seniors.

Promotes Better Posture: Regular practice can strengthen the muscles that support the spine, improving posture and reducing the risk of falls.

Enhances Breath Awareness: The coordinated breath with movement promotes relaxation and helps reduce stress, enhancing overall well-being.

Prepares the Body for Activity: This stretch serves as an excellent warm-up for more strenuous activities, helping to prepare the muscles and joints for movement.

How to Perform the Seated Cat-Cow Stretch
1. Find Your Space
Choose a sturdy chair without arms to ensure you have enough space to move freely. Sit on the edge of the chair with your feet flat on the floor, hip-width apart. Your knees should be directly over your ankles.

2. Position Your Hands
Place your hands on your knees or thighs, palms facing down. This grounding action helps you maintain stability throughout the stretch.

3. Establish Your Breath
Begin by taking a few deep breaths in and out through your nose. Inhale deeply, allowing your belly to expand, and exhale fully, feeling your belly draw back towards your spine. This breathing technique will enhance your connection to the movement.

4. Start the Cat Position
As you exhale, round your back, tucking your chin towards your chest. Imagine you are a cat stretching its back. Engage your abdominal muscles to deepen the stretch in your lower back. Allow your shoulders to relax forward, creating a gentle curve in your spine. Hold this position for a moment, breathing deeply and feeling the stretch in your back.

5. Transition to the Cow Position
As you inhale, arch your back and lift your head and chest. Draw your shoulders back and down, opening up your heart space. Your gaze should gently lift towards the ceiling, creating a gentle curve in your spine. Feel the stretch in your chest and the lengthening in your back.

6. Flow Between the Two Positions
Continue to move between the Cat and Cow positions, coordinating your breath with each movement:

Inhale as you move into Cow, and exhale as you transition back to Cat.

Aim for 5-10 repetitions, maintaining a steady, relaxed breath throughout.

7. Conclude the Stretch

After completing your repetitions, return to a neutral seated position. Take a moment to close your eyes and feel the effects of the stretch. Notice any differences in tension, flexibility, and overall relaxation in your body.

Tips for a Safe and Effective Stretch

Listen to Your Body: It's essential to honor your body's limits. If you experience pain (as opposed to a gentle stretch), ease out of the position and modify your movements.

Modify for Comfort: If you find it challenging to perform the stretch as described, consider using a cushion for additional support or performing the movement with your hands on a sturdy table for stability.

Practice Mindfulness: Pay attention to your breath and movements. This focus enhances the benefits of the stretch and promotes relaxation.

Incorporate the Stretch into Your Routine: Aim to include the Seated Cat-Cow Stretch in your daily routine, whether as part of your morning ritual, during a break in your day, or as a warm-up before other exercises.

The Seated Cat-Cow Stretch is more than just a simple exercise; it's a wonderful way to cultivate body awareness, improve flexibility, and relieve tension. By integrating this stretch into your daily routine, you can enjoy its myriad benefits, paving the way for a more active and fulfilling lifestyle. Remember, consistency is key. Over time, you will likely notice improvements in your mobility, posture, and overall sense of well-being. So find a chair, breathe deeply, and flow into your practice. Your body will thank you!

Seated Forward Bend

The Seated Forward Bend, also known as Paschimottanasana in yoga, is a gentle yet effective stretching exercise that targets the entire back of the body, including the spine, hamstrings, and calves. This pose is particularly beneficial for seniors, as it promotes flexibility, improves posture, and can help alleviate tension in the back and legs. In this guide, we will explore the benefits, proper alignment, modifications, and tips for practicing the Seated Forward Bend safely and effectively.

Benefits of Seated Forward Bend

Enhances Flexibility: The Seated Forward Bend stretches the hamstrings, calves, and lower back, which is essential for maintaining mobility and preventing stiffness as we age.

Improves Posture: By elongating the spine and opening the hips, this pose helps counteract the effects of prolonged sitting and slumping, encouraging better alignment and posture.

Relieves Tension: Sitting in a forward fold can help release tension in the back and shoulders, promoting relaxation and reducing stress levels.

Stimulates Digestive Organs: The forward bend compresses the abdomen gently, stimulating digestive organs and improving circulation to the area.

Calms the Mind: This pose encourages mindfulness and inward focus, helping to calm the nervous system and reduce anxiety.

Prepares for Deeper Stretches: By warming up the hamstrings and lower back, the Seated Forward Bend prepares the body for deeper stretches and more advanced yoga poses.

Getting Started: Setting Up for Seated Forward Bend
Equipment Needed
Yoga Mat: Provides cushioning and stability.
Chair (optional): For added support if sitting on the floor is uncomfortable.
Yoga Strap or Towel: Can be used to assist in reaching the feet if flexibility is limited.
Cushion or Block: For extra support under the hips if needed.
Finding Your Space
Choose a quiet, comfortable space with enough room to stretch out. If you are using a chair, make sure it is sturdy and positioned on a flat surface to prevent any wobbling.

Step-by-Step Instructions for Seated Forward Bend
Step 1: Get into Position
Sit Comfortably: Begin by sitting on the floor with your legs extended straight in front of you. You can also perform this pose seated on the edge of a sturdy chair with your feet flat on the floor.

Posture Alignment: Keep your spine straight and your shoulders relaxed. If you are sitting on the floor and feel tightness in your lower back, place a cushion or yoga block under your hips to elevate your seat.

Step 2: Preparing for the Forward Bend

Engage Your Core: Gently engage your abdominal muscles to support your spine as you prepare to fold forward.

Inhale and Lengthen: Take a deep breath in, lifting your arms overhead. Reach through your fingertips, elongating your spine.

Exhale and Fold: As you exhale, hinge at your hips and slowly fold forward. Imagine bringing your chest towards your thighs rather than rounding your back. If you are sitting in a chair, simply lean slightly forward from your hips, keeping your back straight.

Step 3: Finding Your Depth
Hands Placement: Place your hands on your shins, ankles, or feet, depending on your flexibility. If you can't reach your feet, that's perfectly fine; use a strap around the soles of your feet or hold onto your shins instead.

Relax into the Stretch: Allow your neck to relax and your head to hang heavy. Close your eyes if comfortable and breathe deeply, holding the pose for 30 seconds to a minute, or longer if it feels good.

Stay Aware of Your Body: Keep your shoulders away from your ears and avoid forcing the stretch. It's essential to listen to your body and respect its limits.

Step 4: Coming Out of the Pose
Inhale to Rise: When you're ready to come out of the pose, take a deep breath in. Press your hands gently into your legs, engage your core, and slowly rise back up, returning to a seated position.

Reset Your Posture: Take a moment to sit up tall, rolling your shoulders back and down, and take a few deep breaths to ground yourself.

Modifications and Variations
Using a Chair: If sitting on the floor is uncomfortable, perform the Seated Forward Bend on a chair. Keep your feet flat on the ground, and lean forward from the hips, maintaining a straight back.

With a Strap: If you cannot reach your feet, loop a yoga strap or towel around the balls of your feet. Hold the strap with both hands and gently pull yourself forward.

Bend Your Knees: If your hamstrings are tight, don't hesitate to keep a slight bend in your knees. This adjustment can relieve pressure in the lower back while still providing the benefits of the pose.

Supported Forward Bend: For added support, place a bolster or cushion on your thighs and rest your forehead on it. This variation is particularly soothing and helps alleviate any strain.

Tips for Safe Practice
Listen to Your Body: Always pay attention to how your body feels. If you experience sharp pain or discomfort, ease out of the pose.

Breathe Deeply: Focus on your breath during the pose. Inhale deeply to lengthen the spine, and exhale to deepen the stretch. Breathing can help you relax into the pose and enhance the benefits.

Avoid Overstretching: It's common to want to push for a deeper stretch, but overstretching can lead to injury. Aim for a gentle stretch that feels comfortable and sustainable.

Practice Regularly: To reap the full benefits of the Seated Forward Bend, incorporate it into your regular exercise routine. Practicing consistently can enhance flexibility and strengthen your body over time.

Incorporating Seated Forward Bend into Your Routine
Consider including the Seated Forward Bend in your daily or weekly exercise regimen. You can integrate it into a longer chair yoga session or practice it as a standalone stretch during breaks throughout the day.

The Seated Forward Bend is a powerful yet accessible exercise for seniors looking to improve their flexibility, relieve tension, and enhance their overall well-being. By following the steps outlined in this guide, you can safely incorporate this pose into your fitness routine, gaining the numerous benefits it offers. Remember, yoga is a personal journey; honor your body's needs, and enjoy the process of stretching and strengthening in a way that feels right for you.

Gentle Chair Twist

The Gentle Chair Twist is an excellent exercise for seniors looking to enhance flexibility, improve spinal mobility, and promote relaxation—all while seated safely in a chair. This accessible movement helps to release tension in the spine, shoulders, and hips, making it ideal for those over 60 who may have limited mobility or are new to exercise. In this guide, we'll explore the benefits, step-by-step instructions, variations, and safety tips for performing the Gentle Chair Twist.

Benefits of the Gentle Chair Twist
Improved Spinal Mobility:

The twist encourages rotational movement in the spine, which is often neglected in daily activities. This can help reduce stiffness and improve overall spinal health.
Enhanced Flexibility:

Regular practice of the Gentle Chair Twist can increase flexibility in the back, shoulders, and hips. This is particularly important as we age, as flexibility tends to decrease over time.
Reduced Tension and Stress:

Twisting movements can help alleviate tension in the body, especially in the lower back and hips. This can lead to a sense of relaxation and well-being.
Better Digestion:

Gentle twists stimulate the digestive organs, promoting better digestion and potentially alleviating discomfort related to bloating or constipation.
Improved Posture:

By encouraging spinal alignment and awareness, the Gentle Chair Twist can contribute to better posture, which is crucial for preventing back pain and maintaining balance.
Mind-Body Connection:

The Gentle Chair Twist incorporates breath awareness and mindfulness, fostering a deeper connection between the mind and body, which can enhance overall mental well-being.
Step-by-Step Instructions
Preparation:

Choose the Right Chair:

Select a sturdy chair without arms to allow for easy movement. Ensure the chair is at a height that allows your feet to rest flat on the floor.
Get Comfortable:

Sit up tall in the chair with your back straight. Your feet should be hip-width apart, firmly planted on the ground. Relax your shoulders away from your ears and place your hands on your knees or thighs.

Focus on Your Breath:

Take a few deep breaths to center yourself. Inhale through your nose, filling your lungs, and exhale through your mouth, releasing any tension.
Performing the Gentle Chair Twist:

Starting Position:

Sit comfortably with your feet flat on the floor, spine tall, and shoulders relaxed.
Inhale and Lengthen:

As you inhale, imagine lengthening your spine upward. This prepares your body for the twist.
Initiate the Twist:

On your exhale, gently turn your upper body to the right. Start from your lower back and allow the twist to flow upward through your spine. Keep your hips facing forward and your feet grounded.
Place Your Hand:

As you twist, place your left hand on your right knee or the chair's armrest, if available. Your right hand can rest on the back of the chair or reach out behind you, helping you deepen the twist.
Hold the Position:

Maintain the twist for 3-5 breaths. Focus on breathing deeply into your abdomen, allowing your torso to relax with each exhale. Feel the stretch along your spine and shoulders.
Return to Center:

On an inhale, gently unwind and return to the center. Take a moment to realign your posture and take a few calming breaths.
Repeat on the Other Side:

Exhale and repeat the twist to the left, using the same method. Ensure you maintain your breath and focus throughout the movement.
Complete the Exercise:

Perform the Gentle Chair Twist 3-5 times on each side, allowing yourself to explore the depth of the twist as your body feels comfortable.
Variations and Modifications
Using a Prop:

If you find it difficult to maintain the twist, you can use a small cushion or towel to sit on, providing extra height and support.

Gentle Supported Twist:

For those who need additional support, consider placing a strap or towel around your knees to help guide the twist without straining your body.

Gentle Rotation Without Arm Placement:

If reaching your hands behind is challenging, simply place your hands on your knees and focus on the twist from the lower back, without using your arms for support.

Incorporating Breathing Techniques:

For a more meditative practice, incorporate pranayama (breath control) techniques. Inhale deeply as you lengthen your spine and exhale slowly as you twist, focusing on the sensations in your body.

Safety Tips

Listen to Your Body:

Pay attention to how your body feels during the exercise. If you experience pain, stop and reassess your position. Never force a twist beyond your comfort level.

Avoid Overexertion:

Remember that this exercise is about gentle movement. If you feel dizzy or overly fatigued, pause and take a moment to breathe deeply before continuing.

Consult a Physician:

If you have a history of spinal issues or any health concerns, consult with your physician or a certified fitness professional before attempting the Gentle Chair Twist.

Warm-Up:

Consider performing a gentle warm-up before starting this exercise to prepare your muscles and joints.

Focus on Alignment:

Ensure that your spine is aligned, and avoid collapsing your chest or hunching your shoulders during the twist.

Incorporating the Gentle Chair Twist into Your Routine

The Gentle Chair Twist can be a fantastic addition to your daily routine. Here are a few ideas on how to incorporate it effectively:

Morning Stretch Routine:

Begin your day with the Gentle Chair Twist as part of your morning stretch routine to awaken your body and mind.

During Breaks:

Use the Gentle Chair Twist during breaks throughout your day to relieve tension from prolonged sitting, whether at your desk or while watching television.

Mindfulness Practice:

Combine the twist with mindfulness practices by focusing on your breath and body sensations, allowing it to become a moving meditation.

Pairing with Other Exercises:

Incorporate the Gentle Chair Twist into a larger chair yoga or strength training session to balance your routine with flexibility work.

The Gentle Chair Twist is a simple yet powerful exercise that offers numerous benefits for seniors over 60. With its emphasis on spinal mobility, flexibility, and relaxation, this movement can enhance your overall quality of life. By practicing this exercise regularly, you'll promote better posture, alleviate tension, and cultivate a deeper connection to your body. So, find your chair, take a deep breath, and enjoy the journey of movement and mindfulness through the Gentle Chair Twist!

Seated Mountain Pose

The Seated Mountain Pose, known as Tadasana in Sanskrit, is a foundational yoga posture that promotes stability, strength, and awareness. While it is typically performed in a standing position, the seated variation is especially beneficial for seniors or individuals with limited mobility. This pose allows practitioners to experience the grounding qualities of the Mountain Pose while seated, making it accessible and adaptable.

Benefits of Seated Mountain Pose

Engaging in the Seated Mountain Pose offers numerous benefits:

Improved Posture: This pose encourages proper alignment of the spine, helping to counteract the effects of slouching or hunching over, which is common in sedentary lifestyles.

Strengthens Core Muscles: By engaging the abdominal muscles, the Seated Mountain Pose helps strengthen the core, which is essential for balance and stability.

Enhanced Breathing: This pose promotes deep, mindful breathing, which can reduce stress and anxiety while increasing oxygen flow throughout the body.

Increased Awareness: Practicing Seated Mountain Pose enhances body awareness and mindfulness, allowing individuals to connect with their physical presence and mental state.

Flexibility: Regular practice can improve flexibility in the hips, legs, and lower back, aiding in overall mobility.

Calming the Mind: This pose can serve as a moment of stillness, providing an opportunity to center oneself and reduce mental clutter.

How to Perform Seated Mountain Pose

Step-by-Step Instructions

Preparation:

Find a sturdy chair that offers good support. Ideally, the chair should have a straight back and no armrests to allow for full range of motion.
Sit at the edge of the chair with your feet flat on the floor, hip-width apart. Ensure that your knees are aligned with your ankles.

Posture Alignment:

Place your hands on your thighs, palms facing down or up, depending on your comfort level.
Lengthen your spine by gently rolling your shoulders back and down. Imagine a string pulling the crown of your head toward the ceiling. Your neck should be in line with your spine.
Engage your abdominal muscles slightly to support your lower back without tensing.

Foot Placement:

Distribute your weight evenly across your feet. Press firmly into the floor with all four corners of your feet—the base of the big toe, the base of the little toe, and the heel.

Feel the connection of your feet to the ground, allowing you to sense stability.
Breathing:

Close your eyes or soften your gaze to minimize distractions. Begin to take deep, slow breaths in through your nose, allowing your abdomen to expand fully.

As you exhale, feel your body soften and release any tension. Continue to breathe deeply, focusing on your breath and the sensations within your body.

Duration:

Hold the pose for 30 seconds to a minute, or longer if comfortable. Use this time to cultivate a sense of inner calm and focus.
Releasing the Pose:

To exit the pose, gently open your eyes, if closed, and take a few deep breaths. Begin to shift your awareness back to the room around you.

Slowly bring your hands back to your thighs or at your heart center. Gently roll your shoulders back and down, then return to your regular seated position.

Common Mistakes to Avoid

Slouching or Leaning Back: Ensure that you maintain an upright posture. Avoid leaning against the back of the chair, as this can reduce the effectiveness of the pose.

Holding Your Breath: Remember to breathe deeply and evenly. Holding your breath can create tension in the body and reduce the calming benefits of the pose.

Over-Tensing Muscles: While it's important to engage your core and maintain a strong posture, avoid excessive tension. The goal is to feel both strength and relaxation.
Modifications and Variations

The Seated Mountain Pose can be easily modified to suit individual needs:

Use of Props: If you have difficulty sitting upright, consider using a cushion or folded blanket to elevate your hips, which can help align your spine more comfortably.

Chair with Armrests: If balance is an issue, using a chair with armrests can provide additional support. Just ensure you don't rely on them too heavily.

Hands at Heart Center: Instead of resting your hands on your thighs, bring them together at your heart center. This can enhance your sense of focus and grounding.

Integrating Seated Mountain Pose into

Your Routine

To maximize the benefits of the Seated Mountain Pose, consider integrating it into your daily routine:

Morning Routine: Start your day with a few minutes in Seated Mountain Pose to awaken your body and mind. Set a positive intention for the day ahead.

Midday Break: Take a break during your day to practice the pose. This can help clear your mind and reduce stress, making it easier to refocus on tasks.

Pre-Bedtime Wind Down: Incorporate Seated Mountain Pose into your evening routine to calm your mind and prepare for restful sleep.

Mindfulness Practice: Use this pose as part of a mindfulness or meditation session. Focus on your breath and the sensations in your body to deepen your practice.

The Seated Mountain Pose is a powerful yet simple exercise that offers numerous benefits for seniors and individuals of all fitness levels. By incorporating this pose into your routine, you can improve your posture, increase flexibility, and cultivate a deeper mind-body connection.

Remember, the key to a successful practice is consistency and mindfulness. Listen to your body, honor your limits, and enjoy the journey toward enhanced strength, flexibility, and overall well-being. Whether you're just starting your fitness journey or looking to maintain your current health, the Seated Mountain Pose is an excellent addition to your daily routine.

Chair Yoga Flow: A 10-Minute Routine to Start Your Day

As we age, maintaining flexibility, strength, and balance becomes increasingly important. Chair yoga is an excellent way to achieve these goals while ensuring safety and accessibility for seniors. In this guide, we'll walk through a comprehensive 10-minute chair yoga flow designed to energize your morning, enhance your flexibility, and set a positive tone for the day ahead.

The Benefits of Chair Yoga
Before diving into our routine, let's take a moment to appreciate why chair yoga is so beneficial:

Accessibility: Chair yoga can be practiced by individuals with limited mobility or balance issues, allowing everyone to experience the benefits of yoga.

Flexibility: Regular practice helps increase flexibility in joints and muscles, which is essential for maintaining mobility and reducing the risk of injuries.

Strength: Many chair yoga poses engage different muscle groups, helping to build strength without the strain of traditional weightlifting.

Mindfulness: The practice encourages deep breathing and focus, promoting mental clarity and reducing stress.

Convenience: You can practice chair yoga in the comfort of your home, making it a perfect addition to your morning routine.

Preparing for Your Chair Yoga Flow
Setting Up Your Space

Choose a Comfortable Chair: Opt for a sturdy chair without arms to allow for a full range of motion. Make sure it's at a height where your feet can rest flat on the floor.

Create a Calm Environment: Find a quiet space where you won't be disturbed. Consider soft lighting, and if you enjoy music, play some calming tunes in the background.

Dress Comfortably: Wear loose, breathable clothing that allows for easy movement. Avoid restrictive fabrics that could hinder your flow.

Gather Props: You might want a yoga mat to place under your chair for extra stability, a water bottle to stay hydrated, and a small towel to wipe off any perspiration.

Your 10-Minute Chair Yoga Routine
Warm-Up (2 minutes)

Start by preparing your body for movement with some gentle stretches.

Seated Cat-Cow Stretch

Sit up tall in your chair with your feet flat on the ground.
Place your hands on your knees.
Inhale as you arch your back, lifting your chest and looking slightly upward (Cow Pose).
Exhale as you round your back, tucking your chin towards your chest (Cat Pose).
Repeat this sequence for 5 breaths, allowing your spine to articulate gently.

Neck Rolls

Sit comfortably with your back straight.
Drop your right ear towards your right shoulder and let your head roll gently forward and then to the left.
Complete the roll by bringing your left ear to your left shoulder, then back to center.
Do this for 3 complete rolls in one direction, then switch to the other direction.
Main Flow (6 minutes)

Now, we'll transition into the main flow of poses that focus on flexibility and strength.

Seated Mountain Pose (1 minute)

Sit up tall with your feet hip-width apart and grounded.
Place your hands on your thighs, palms facing up.
Close your eyes and take five deep breaths, feeling your spine lengthen with each inhale. Focus on grounding your feet and lifting through the crown of your head.
Seated Forward Bend (1 minute)

Inhale and raise your arms overhead, stretching your sides.
Exhale as you hinge at your hips, lowering your torso toward your knees while keeping your back straight.
Let your hands rest on your shins or thighs. Hold for five deep breaths, feeling the stretch in your back and hamstrings.
Seated Side Stretch (1 minute)

Return to an upright position and place your right hand on the seat of your chair.
Inhale and raise your left arm overhead.
Exhale as you lean to the right, feeling a stretch along your left side. Hold for three deep breaths.
Inhale to return to center and switch sides.
Chair Twist (1 minute)

Sit tall and place your right hand on the back of the chair for support.
Inhale as you lengthen your spine, and exhale as you gently twist to the right, looking over your shoulder.
Hold for five breaths, feeling the gentle rotation in your spine.
Inhale to return to center and repeat on the left side.
Seated Leg Lifts (1 minute)

Sit at the edge of your chair with your feet flat on the ground.

Inhale as you lift your right leg straight out in front of you, keeping your knee straight.
Exhale as you lower it back down without letting your foot touch the floor.
Repeat for five reps, then switch to the left leg.
Seated Calf Raises (1 minute)

Sit tall and place your feet flat on the ground.
Inhale as you rise up onto your toes, engaging your calf muscles.
Exhale as you lower back down.
Repeat this movement for 10 reps, feeling the muscles in your lower legs activate.
Cool Down (2 minutes)

Finish your routine with some gentle stretches and relaxation.

Seated Figure Four Stretch (1 minute)

Sit tall and place your right ankle over your left knee.
Gently press down on your right knee to deepen the stretch in your hip.
Lean forward slightly to increase the stretch. Hold for five breaths.
Switch sides and repeat.
Seated Relaxation (1 minute)

Sit comfortably with your feet flat on the ground.
Place your hands on your knees and close your eyes.
Take five deep breaths, allowing your body to relax and settle. Focus on how you feel after this practice.
Chair yoga is an excellent way to start your day, providing a gentle yet effective way to increase flexibility, strength, and mindfulness. By incorporating this 10-minute routine into your morning, you'll likely notice improvements in your physical capabilities, a reduction in stress, and an overall sense of well-being.

Remember, the key to any exercise routine is consistency. Aim to practice this flow daily or several times a week to reap the full benefits. As you become more comfortable, feel free to explore other chair yoga poses and integrate them into your routine. Here's to a healthier, happier you!

Chapter 4: Strength Training with Chairs and Light Weights

Why Strength Training is Vital After 60

As we age, our bodies undergo a series of transformations that can impact our strength, mobility, and overall quality of life. By the time we reach our 60s, it's not uncommon to experience a gradual decline in muscle mass, bone density, and physical function. This phenomenon, often referred to as sarcopenia, is a natural part of the aging process. However, it doesn't have to dictate our health or well-being in our later years. Strength training emerges as a vital component for seniors, offering numerous benefits that enhance not only physical capabilities but also mental and emotional health.

Understanding Muscle Loss and Its Implications
Research indicates that individuals can lose approximately 3% to 5% of their muscle mass per decade after the age of 30, and this rate accelerates after 60. This loss of muscle can lead to decreased strength, reduced mobility, and an increased risk of falls. Furthermore, the repercussions extend beyond mere physical limitations. A reduction in strength can lead to a decline in independence, making everyday activities—like climbing stairs, carrying groceries, or even standing up from a chair—more challenging.

Muscle strength is crucial for supporting joints and maintaining proper posture, both of which can help prevent injuries. Additionally, strength training can significantly impact bone density. As we age, our bones naturally become weaker, making us more susceptible to fractures. Engaging in regular resistance exercises helps stimulate bone formation and slows down the loss of bone density, which is particularly important for women who are at a higher risk for osteoporosis.

The Benefits of Strength Training for Seniors
Enhancing Functional Fitness:
Strength training focuses on building muscle strength, which translates directly into functional fitness. This means that everyday tasks become easier and less tiring. Lifting objects, getting up from a seated position, and even walking can become more manageable with increased strength. Improved functional fitness directly contributes to maintaining independence in later years.

Boosting Metabolism:
Muscle tissue is metabolically active, meaning that the more muscle you have, the more calories your body burns at rest. This is particularly beneficial for seniors looking to manage their weight.

Engaging in regular strength training can help counteract the slower metabolism that often accompanies aging, making it easier to maintain a healthy weight.

Improving Balance and Stability:
One of the most significant risks for seniors is falls. Strength training enhances balance by developing the muscles that support stability. Stronger muscles, particularly in the lower body, help prevent falls and the injuries that can accompany them, such as fractures. Exercises like squats, lunges, and step-ups specifically target balance and coordination.

Enhancing Mental Health:
The psychological benefits of strength training are equally important. Exercise, including strength training, releases endorphins, which are chemicals in the brain that promote a sense of well-being. This can help combat feelings of anxiety and depression, common challenges faced by many older adults. Additionally, achieving fitness goals—no matter how small—can significantly boost self-esteem and confidence.

Promoting Healthy Aging:
Strength training has been linked to a range of health benefits that contribute to overall well-being. Regular resistance exercise can lower the risk of chronic diseases, improve cardiovascular health, and enhance insulin sensitivity. This is particularly important for seniors at risk of diabetes or heart disease. Moreover, strength training can help manage chronic pain conditions, such as arthritis, by improving joint function and reducing stiffness.

Social Engagement and Motivation:
Participating in group strength training classes or finding a workout buddy can provide essential social interaction. This can help combat loneliness and isolation, which can be significant issues for seniors. A supportive community encourages motivation and accountability, making it easier to stick to a regular exercise routine.

Getting Started with Strength Training
If you're new to strength training or returning after a long break, it's essential to approach it safely and gradually. Here are some key points to consider:

Consult with a Professional:
Before starting any exercise program, particularly strength training, consult with a healthcare provider or a fitness professional experienced in working with seniors. They can help assess your current fitness level and any medical conditions that might affect your exercise routine.

Start Slow:

Begin with light weights or resistance bands and focus on proper form and technique. Bodyweight exercises, such as squats and push-ups, can also be effective for building strength without added resistance. Gradually increase the weight and intensity as your strength improves.

Focus on Major Muscle Groups:
Aim to include exercises that target all major muscle groups: legs, back, chest, arms, and core. This can help ensure balanced strength development and reduce the risk of injury.

Incorporate Flexibility and Balance Training:
Combine strength training with flexibility and balance exercises. This holistic approach will enhance overall fitness and further reduce the risk of falls. Activities like yoga or Tai Chi can be excellent complements to strength training.

Create a Routine:
Establish a consistent routine that fits your lifestyle. Aim for at least two to three strength training sessions per week, with rest days in between to allow your muscles to recover.

Listen to Your Body:
Pay attention to how your body feels during and after workouts. Some soreness is normal, but sharp pain is not. Adjust your routine as necessary and seek professional guidance if you experience discomfort.

Strength training is not just for bodybuilders or younger athletes; it is an essential practice for seniors that can significantly enhance quality of life. By incorporating strength training into your weekly routine, you can combat muscle loss, maintain independence, improve balance, and promote overall health. The key is to start slowly, be consistent, and enjoy the journey towards greater strength and vitality. Embracing strength training after 60 is a powerful way to take charge of your health and embrace the possibilities of aging with confidence and grace.

How to Use Weights Safely

As a fitness instructor with years of experience working with seniors, I understand that using weights can be daunting for many. The good news is that with the right approach, strength training can be an incredibly beneficial part of your fitness routine. This guide will walk you through everything you need to know to use weights safely and effectively, empowering you to enhance your strength, improve your mobility, and maintain your independence as you age.

Understanding the Benefits of Strength Training

Before we delve into the specifics of using weights safely, let's briefly explore the benefits of strength training, particularly for those over 60. Engaging in regular strength training:

Improves Muscle Mass and Strength: As we age, we naturally lose muscle mass, a process known as sarcopenia. Strength training helps counteract this by stimulating muscle growth and improving overall strength, making everyday activities easier and reducing the risk of falls.

Enhances Bone Density: Resistance training helps increase bone density, which is crucial for preventing osteoporosis and fractures. Stronger bones support your overall skeletal structure, providing better stability.

Boosts Metabolism: Building muscle through strength training increases your resting metabolic rate. This means your body will burn more calories at rest, which can assist in weight management.

Improves Joint Health: Strengthening the muscles around your joints can help stabilize them, reducing pain and improving overall mobility. This is especially beneficial for seniors who may experience joint pain from arthritis or other conditions.

Supports Mental Health: Engaging in regular exercise, including strength training, has been shown to reduce symptoms of depression and anxiety, boost mood, and enhance cognitive function.

Getting Started: Consult Your Doctor
Before starting any new exercise regimen, especially if you have existing health concerns, it's essential to consult your healthcare provider. They can provide guidance based on your individual health status and help you understand any limitations or considerations you should keep in mind while exercising.

Choosing the Right Weights
When it comes to selecting weights, here are some important factors to consider:

Start Light: If you are new to strength training or haven't exercised in a while, it's best to start with light weights. This could be 1 to 5-pound dumbbells, resistance bands, or even your body weight. The goal is to learn proper form and technique without straining your muscles.

Choose Adjustable Weights: If possible, use adjustable weights or resistance bands that allow you to modify the intensity of your workout. This flexibility enables you to gradually increase resistance as you build strength.

Listen to Your Body: Pay attention to how your body feels. If a weight feels too heavy, it probably is. It's essential to feel challenged but not overwhelmed. The right weight will allow you to perform exercises with good form for the entire set.

Proper Techniques for Weight Training
Using weights safely is not just about choosing the right amount; it's also about mastering proper techniques to prevent injury. Here are some key tips to ensure safe weight training:

Warm Up Properly: Always start your workout with a warm-up to prepare your muscles and joints for activity. This can include light cardio (such as marching in place or walking) and dynamic stretches that mimic the movements you'll perform during your workout.

Focus on Form: Proper form is crucial when using weights. Here are some pointers:

Alignment: Keep your spine neutral, with your shoulders back and down, and avoid arching your back.
Movement: Control your movements, avoiding swinging or jerking motions. Perform exercises slowly and deliberately.
Breathing: Breathe out when you lift (the exertion phase) and breathe in when you lower the weight. This helps maintain core stability.
Engage Your Core: Before lifting weights, engage your core muscles by drawing your navel in towards your spine. This stabilizes your body and protects your back during weight-bearing exercises.

Use a Full Range of Motion: Whenever possible, perform exercises through a full range of motion. This means fully extending and contracting the muscles to maximize the benefits of each exercise.

Avoid Holding Your Breath: Proper breathing is vital. Holding your breath can increase blood pressure and lead to dizziness. Maintain a steady breath throughout your exercises.

Common Exercises and Safety Tips
Here are some safe and effective weight training exercises that seniors can perform using weights or resistance bands, along with safety tips for each:

1. Seated Bicep Curls
How to Perform: Sit in a sturdy chair with your feet flat on the floor. Hold a dumbbell in each hand with your arms at your sides. Slowly curl the weights towards your shoulders while keeping your elbows close to your body. Lower back down to the starting position.

Safety Tips: Keep your back straight and avoid leaning forward. Start with a light weight to master the motion.

2. Seated Shoulder Press

How to Perform: Sit in a chair with a dumbbell in each hand at shoulder height, palms facing forward. Press the weights overhead until your arms are fully extended, then lower them back to shoulder height.

Safety Tips: Ensure your feet are flat on the ground and your back is supported by the chair. Avoid arching your back during the lift.

3. Standing Leg Lifts

How to Perform: Stand behind a chair and hold onto it for support. Slowly lift one leg out to the side, keeping your body straight. Hold for a moment, then lower it back down. Repeat on the other side.

Safety Tips: Focus on balance; if you feel unsteady, perform the exercise seated. Use light ankle weights or no weights at all if you're just starting.

4. Chair-Assisted Squats

How to Perform: Stand in front of a sturdy chair, feet shoulder-width apart. Lower yourself as if you are going to sit down, but stop just above the chair, then return to standing.

Safety Tips: Keep your knees aligned with your toes and do not let them extend past your toes. If needed, use a lightweight dumbbell in one hand for added resistance while holding the chair with the other hand.

5. Seated Row with Resistance Bands

How to Perform: Sit with your legs extended, loop a resistance band around your feet, and hold the ends in your hands. Pull the band towards your torso, squeezing your shoulder blades together, then release slowly.

Safety Tips: Keep your back straight and avoid rounding your shoulders. Ensure the band is securely anchored and not frayed.

Cool Down and Stretch

After your strength training session, it's crucial to cool down and stretch to promote recovery and flexibility. Here's a simple cool-down routine:

Gentle Walking: Spend 5 minutes walking slowly to lower your heart rate.

Static Stretches: Hold each stretch for 15-30 seconds:

Hamstring Stretch: While seated, extend one leg and reach towards your toes.

Shoulder Stretch: Bring one arm across your body and hold it with the opposite hand.

Neck Stretch: Gently tilt your head to one side, bringing your ear towards your shoulder.

Listening to Your Body: Know When to Stop

Pay close attention to your body during and after your workout. It's normal to feel some soreness, but you should never feel pain. If you experience sharp or sudden pain, dizziness, or shortness of breath, stop exercising immediately and consult your healthcare provider. Remember that progress takes time; be patient and focus on consistency rather than intensity.

Conclusion

Using weights safely is a vital part of any fitness routine, especially for seniors looking to improve their strength and flexibility. By starting with light weights, mastering proper techniques, and listening to your body, you can enjoy the numerous benefits of strength training without the risk of injury. Embrace this empowering journey toward better health and fitness, and remember: it's never too late to start! With dedication and the right approach, you can enhance your quality of life and maintain your independence for years to come.

Resources

Consider enrolling in a local exercise class specifically designed for seniors to gain confidence and receive professional guidance.

Many online platforms offer virtual classes tailored to seniors, making it easy to follow along from the comfort of your home.

Invest in instructional videos or apps that emphasize proper techniques for strength training.

By following these guidelines, you will be well-equipped to safely incorporate weights into your exercise routine, fostering strength, flexibility, and overall well-being in your golden years.

Chair-Based Strength Exercises

As we age, maintaining strength becomes essential for daily activities, enhancing mobility, and ensuring independence. Chair-based strength exercises are an excellent way for seniors to engage in resistance training safely and effectively. These exercises not only help in building muscle strength but also improve balance, coordination, and overall functional fitness. We'll delve into various chair-based strength exercises, explore their benefits, and provide step-by-step instructions to ensure you perform them safely and effectively.

Why Chair-Based Strength Exercises?

Safety and Accessibility: Chairs provide stability and support, reducing the risk of falls or injuries, which can be a concern for older adults.

Flexibility of Location: These exercises can be performed at home, in community centers, or anywhere with a sturdy chair, making it convenient to fit into your routine.

Engagement of Multiple Muscle Groups: Many chair exercises engage several muscle groups simultaneously, promoting overall strength and functionality.

Adaptability: Exercises can be modified for various fitness levels, ensuring that everyone can participate, whether you are a beginner or have been exercising for years.

Getting Started: Preparing for Chair-Based Strength Training

Before diving into specific exercises, it's crucial to prepare your body. Follow these steps to ensure a safe and effective workout session:

Consult with Your Doctor: Always seek medical advice before starting any exercise program, especially if you have existing health conditions.

Warm-Up: Begin with a gentle warm-up to get your blood flowing and your muscles ready. A simple warm-up could include seated marches, arm circles, or gentle torso twists for about 5-10 minutes.

Choose the Right Chair: Select a sturdy chair without arms that provides good support. The height should allow your feet to rest flat on the ground when seated.

Have Equipment Ready: If possible, use light weights (1-5 pounds), resistance bands, or household items like water bottles or cans. Ensure your space is clear of obstacles to prevent falls.

Essential Chair-Based Strength Exercises

Here's a selection of effective chair-based strength exercises designed to target various muscle groups:

1. Seated Leg Lifts

Muscle Groups: Quadriceps, hip flexors, and core.

Instructions:

Sit up straight in your chair, with your back against the backrest and feet flat on the floor.
Slowly extend your right leg out in front of you until it is straight and parallel to the ground.
Hold for a count of 3, then lower it back to the starting position.
Repeat for 10-15 repetitions, then switch to the left leg.

Tips:

Engage your core throughout the movement to maintain balance.
For an added challenge, you can hold a light weight on your extended leg.

2. Chair-Assisted Squats

Muscle Groups: Quadriceps, hamstrings, glutes, and lower back.

Instructions:

Stand in front of your chair with feet shoulder-width apart.
Slowly lower your body as if you are going to sit down, keeping your weight in your heels and chest up.
Stop just above the seat of the chair (or lightly touch it) and hold for a moment.
Rise back to standing and repeat for 10-15 repetitions.

Tips:

Keep your knees aligned with your toes to prevent strain.

Use the chair for support but try to minimize contact to enhance muscle engagement.

3. Seated Bicep Curls

Muscle Groups: Biceps and forearms.

Instructions:

Sit up straight in your chair with a weight in each hand (or water bottles).
Start with your arms at your sides, palms facing forward.
Slowly curl the weights toward your shoulders, keeping your elbows close to your body.
Lower the weights back to the starting position. Repeat for 10-15 repetitions.

Tips:

Focus on controlled movements rather than speed to maximize muscle engagement.
Ensure that your wrists are straight and not bent during the curls.

4. Overhead Press

Muscle Groups: Shoulders, triceps, and upper back.

Instructions:

Sit up straight with a weight in each hand at shoulder height, palms facing forward.
Press the weights overhead until your arms are fully extended.
Lower the weights back to shoulder height. Repeat for 10-15 repetitions.

Tips:

Avoid arching your back; engage your core for support.
Start with lighter weights if you're new to this exercise.

5. Seated Marches

Muscle Groups: Hip flexors, quadriceps, and core.

Instructions:

Sit tall in your chair with feet flat on the floor.
Lift your right knee toward your chest while keeping your left foot on the ground.
Lower your right leg and lift your left knee. Continue alternating for 10-15 repetitions per leg.

Tips:

Use your arms to mimic a marching motion for added intensity.
Keep your movements slow and controlled to focus on muscle engagement.

6. Seated Side Leg Raises

Muscle Groups: Hip abductors and outer thighs.

Instructions:

Sit at the edge of your chair with your feet flat on the floor.
Extend your right leg out to the side, keeping it straight and in line with your hip.
Hold for a moment before lowering it back to the starting position. Repeat for 10-15 repetitions and then switch legs.
Tips:

Keep your torso upright to maintain balance.
You can add ankle weights for an extra challenge as you become stronger.
Creating Your Routine
To maximize the benefits of chair-based strength exercises, aim for 2-3 sessions per week. Here's a sample routine to get you started:

Warm-Up: 5-10 minutes of gentle movements.
Exercises:
Seated Leg Lifts: 2 sets of 10-15 reps (each leg)
Chair-Assisted Squats: 2 sets of 10-15 reps
Seated Bicep Curls: 2 sets of 10-15 reps
Overhead Press: 2 sets of 10-15 reps
Seated Marches: 2 sets of 10-15 reps (each leg)
Seated Side Leg Raises: 2 sets of 10-15 reps (each leg)
Cool Down: 5-10 minutes of stretching, focusing on the legs, arms, and back.
Staying Motivated and Safe
Track Your Progress: Keep a journal of your workouts, noting repetitions, weights used, and how you feel after each session. This can help you see your improvements over time and stay motivated.
Listen to Your Body: It's essential to be mindful of how your body responds to each exercise. If you experience pain (not to be confused with muscle fatigue), stop immediately and consult with a healthcare professional.
Invite a Buddy: Exercising with a friend or family member can make your workouts more enjoyable and keep you accountable.

Chair-based strength exercises provide a practical and effective way for seniors to enhance their strength, flexibility, and overall fitness. By incorporating these exercises into your weekly routine, you'll not only improve your physical health but also boost your confidence and independence in daily activities. Remember, the journey to strength and wellness is a marathon, not a sprint. Celebrate every small victory, and keep moving forward, one chair-based exercise at a time!

Seated Leg Lifts

As we age, maintaining mobility and strength becomes increasingly important. One of the most effective exercises that can be performed while seated is the seated leg lift. This simple yet powerful movement targets the hip flexors, quadriceps, and core muscles, promoting strength, stability, and flexibility. Additionally, seated leg lifts are particularly beneficial for seniors, as they can be performed in a chair, reducing the risk of falls and providing a safe way to enhance lower body strength.

Benefits of Seated Leg Lifts
Before diving into the details of how to perform seated leg lifts, let's discuss why this exercise is a fantastic addition to any fitness routine, especially for seniors:

Improved Muscle Strength: Seated leg lifts primarily engage the quadriceps, the large muscles on the front of the thigh. Strengthening these muscles helps support knee function, improve stability, and enhance overall mobility.

Enhanced Core Stability: While performing leg lifts, your core muscles work to stabilize your body. A strong core is essential for maintaining balance and reducing the risk of falls, which is crucial for seniors.

Increased Flexibility: This exercise promotes flexibility in the hips and legs, allowing for greater ease of movement in daily activities such as walking, climbing stairs, or getting in and out of a car.

Low Impact: Seated leg lifts are a low-impact exercise, making them suitable for individuals with joint pain or arthritis. The seated position reduces strain on the knees and lower back, allowing you to focus on strengthening without discomfort.

Convenience: This exercise can be performed almost anywhere, whether at home, in a gym, or even at a community center. All you need is a sturdy chair with no arms, making it accessible for everyone.

How to Perform Seated Leg Lifts
Preparation
Choose the Right Chair: Select a sturdy chair without arms that allows you to sit comfortably with your feet flat on the floor. Ensure that the chair is stable and will not wobble during the exercise.

Sit Properly: Sit up straight in the chair, with your back against the seat. Keep your shoulders relaxed and your feet hip-width apart, flat on the floor.

Engage Your Core: Before you begin the exercise, engage your abdominal muscles. Imagine pulling your belly button toward your spine. This engagement will help support your lower back throughout the movement.

Execution of Seated Leg Lifts
Lift One Leg: Slowly extend your right leg out in front of you. Keep your knee straight, and raise your leg until it is parallel to the floor or as high as you comfortably can. Be mindful of your posture; maintain an upright position throughout the movement.

Hold the Position: Once your leg is lifted, hold it in position for a count of 3 to 5 seconds. During this hold, focus on squeezing your quadriceps and maintaining core engagement.

Lower Your Leg: Gradually lower your right leg back down to the starting position without letting your foot touch the floor. This helps keep the muscles engaged and provides a continuous challenge.

Repeat: Perform 10 to 15 repetitions with your right leg. After completing the set, switch to your left leg and repeat the same steps.

Tips for Proper Form
Breathe: Remember to breathe throughout the exercise. Inhale as you lift your leg and exhale as you lower it back down.
Avoid Overexertion: Only lift your leg as high as you can without causing strain. If you feel any discomfort, lower the height of your lift or take a break.
Use Your Arms: For added support, you can place your hands on the sides of the chair or hold onto the seat. This will help maintain balance as you perform the exercise.
Stay Mindful: Focus on your movements. Concentrate on the muscles you are engaging, which enhances the effectiveness of the exercise.
Variations and Modifications
As you become more comfortable with seated leg lifts, you may want to explore variations to further challenge your muscles:

Add Ankle Weights: Once you feel confident in your strength, consider using ankle weights to increase the intensity of the exercise. Start with light weights and gradually increase as your strength improves.

Heel and Toe Raises: Combine seated leg lifts with heel and toe raises. After lifting your leg, flex your foot to point your toes away from you and then bring them back toward your body. This adds a greater range of motion and works additional muscles.

Resistance Bands: If you have resistance bands, you can loop one around your feet while seated. This will provide extra resistance when lifting your leg, further enhancing muscle strength.

Incorporate Arm Movements: To engage your upper body, try incorporating arm movements while performing leg lifts. For instance, raise your arms overhead while lifting your leg, or perform bicep curls with light weights as you lift your legs.

Incorporating Seated Leg Lifts into Your Routine
To maximize the benefits of seated leg lifts, consider incorporating them into a comprehensive exercise routine. Here's a simple plan:

Warm-Up: Always start with a gentle warm-up to prepare your muscles. This could include simple neck rolls, shoulder circles, and light seated twists.

Seated Leg Lifts: Perform 2 to 3 sets of 10 to 15 repetitions for each leg.

Complementary Exercises: Follow up with additional chair exercises such as seated arm curls, seated marching, and seated side leg lifts to create a well-rounded routine.

Cool Down: End your workout with some gentle stretching. Focus on your quadriceps, hamstrings, and hip flexors to maintain flexibility.

Seated leg lifts are an excellent exercise for seniors looking to enhance their strength, flexibility, and overall fitness. They are easy to perform, adaptable to various fitness levels, and provide a multitude of benefits without the risk of injury. By incorporating seated leg lifts into your exercise routine, you'll not only improve your physical health but also enhance your quality of life, allowing you to engage in daily activities with greater ease and confidence.

As with any exercise program, be sure to listen to your body and consult with a healthcare provider before starting new workouts, especially if you have existing health concerns. Start slowly, stay consistent, and enjoy the journey to a stronger, healthier you!

Chair-Assisted Squats

Chair-assisted squats are an excellent exercise option for seniors looking to improve their strength, balance, and overall fitness. This exercise is particularly beneficial because it allows individuals to work on their lower body strength while providing the safety and support of a chair. Whether you are just starting your fitness journey or looking to incorporate more strength training into your routine, chair-assisted squats can be an integral part of your regimen.

Why Chair-Assisted Squats?
Before diving into the details of how to perform chair-assisted squats, let's explore the numerous benefits this exercise offers:

Enhanced Leg Strength: Squats primarily target the quadriceps, hamstrings, and glutes, which are crucial for everyday activities like walking, climbing stairs, and getting in and out of chairs. Strengthening these muscles can help improve your overall mobility.

Improved Balance and Stability: Regular practice of chair-assisted squats helps to enhance your balance and coordination. This is especially important as we age, as balance issues can lead to falls and injuries.

Joint Health: Squats, when performed correctly, can help increase flexibility in the hips and knees. This is vital for maintaining joint health and preventing stiffness.

Functional Fitness: Chair-assisted squats mimic movements that we do in daily life. By practicing these squats, you prepare your body for activities like sitting down and standing up, which can make daily tasks feel easier and more manageable.

Accessibility: Using a chair for support makes squats accessible for individuals with varying fitness levels, especially those who may not be able to perform traditional squats due to limited strength or balance issues.

Preparing for Chair-Assisted Squats
1. Choose the Right Chair:

Select a sturdy chair without wheels that can support your weight. Ideally, the seat height should be at a level that allows your feet to touch the ground when seated.
Ensure that the chair is stable and placed against a wall or on a non-slippery surface to prevent movement during the exercise.
2. Dress Comfortably:

Wear comfortable clothing that allows for freedom of movement. Opt for supportive shoes with a good grip to enhance stability during the squats.

3. Warm-Up:

It's essential to warm up your body before starting any exercise. Perform light cardio activities like walking or marching in place for 5–10 minutes. Follow this with dynamic stretches focusing on your legs and hips, such as leg swings and gentle side bends.

How to Perform Chair-Assisted Squats

Now that you are prepared, it's time to learn how to execute chair-assisted squats effectively.

1. Starting Position:

Stand in front of the chair, facing away from it. Your feet should be shoulder-width apart, and your toes should point slightly outward.

Engage your core by pulling your belly button toward your spine to provide stability. This will help support your lower back throughout the exercise.

2. Lowering into the Squat:

Begin by bending your knees and pushing your hips back as if you are going to sit down. Keep your weight in your heels and your chest lifted.

Reach back with your hands to hold onto the chair's armrests or seat for support. This will help maintain balance and provide assistance as you lower your body.

Aim to lower your body until your thighs are parallel to the ground, or as far as is comfortable for you. Ensure that your knees do not extend beyond your toes to prevent strain.

3. Holding the Position:

Pause in the squat position for a moment, taking a deep breath. This is a good time to assess how your body feels. If you experience any discomfort in your knees or back, adjust your position slightly or limit your range of motion.

4. Rising Back Up:

To rise back to a standing position, press through your heels, engaging your glutes and thighs.

Use your arms to assist by pushing off the chair if needed. Keep your core engaged and maintain an upright posture as you stand.

5. Repeat:

Aim for 10-15 repetitions, resting for 30 seconds to a minute between sets. As you become more comfortable with the movement, you can gradually increase the number of repetitions or sets.

Modifications and Variations

Chair-assisted squats can be easily modified to suit your fitness level. Here are some variations you might consider:

Partial Squats: If lowering all the way to parallel is too challenging, perform partial squats, lowering yourself only as far as is comfortable.
Single-Leg Squats: Once you feel confident, you can try a single-leg squat by lifting one leg off the ground while performing the squat with the other leg, using the chair for balance.
Weighted Squats: As your strength improves, consider holding light weights (like water bottles or small dumbbells) in your hands to increase resistance.
Safety Tips
Always listen to your body. If you feel pain (not to be confused with muscle fatigue), stop the exercise immediately.
Focus on maintaining good form. It's better to perform fewer repetitions correctly than to do more with poor technique.
Consider consulting with a fitness professional or physical therapist before beginning any new exercise routine, especially if you have existing health conditions or concerns.
Incorporating Chair-Assisted Squats into Your Routine
Aim to include chair-assisted squats in your exercise regimen at least 2-3 times a week. They can be part of a larger strength training routine or a stand-alone exercise session. Pair them with upper body exercises or stretching for a complete workout.

Sample Routine:

Warm-Up: 5-10 minutes of light cardio.
Chair-Assisted Squats: 2-3 sets of 10-15 repetitions.
Upper Body Strength Exercises (e.g., seated bicep curls or shoulder presses): 2 sets of 10-15 repetitions each.
Cool Down: Gentle stretching for your legs, hips, and back.

Chair-assisted squats are a powerful yet gentle way for seniors to build strength, enhance balance, and improve overall functionality. With practice, this exercise can contribute significantly to your fitness journey, helping you feel more confident and capable in your daily activities. Remember to focus on form, progress at your own pace, and most importantly, enjoy the process of becoming stronger and healthier!

Bicep Curls with Light Weights

Bicep curls are one of the most recognized and effective exercises for strengthening the arms, specifically targeting the biceps brachii. For seniors, particularly those over 60, incorporating light weights into your fitness routine can yield significant benefits, including improved muscle strength, enhanced functional mobility, and increased independence in daily activities. This guide will walk you through the importance of bicep curls, proper technique, modifications, and tips for incorporating them into your workout routine.

The Importance of Bicep Curls for Seniors
As we age, maintaining muscle mass and strength becomes crucial. Sarcopenia, the gradual loss of muscle mass and strength that occurs with aging, can lead to decreased mobility and increased risk of falls. Here's why bicep curls are particularly beneficial:

Strengthening Arm Muscles: Bicep curls specifically target the biceps, which are essential for various daily tasks such as lifting, carrying, and reaching.

Improved Functional Fitness: Stronger arms translate to improved performance in everyday activities, like grocery shopping, lifting grandchildren, or even getting up from a seated position.

Injury Prevention: Strengthening the muscles around your joints can provide better support, reducing the risk of injuries, especially in the shoulders and elbows.

Enhanced Balance and Stability: Strong arm muscles contribute to overall body strength, which is essential for maintaining balance and stability.

Boosting Metabolism: While light weights may not be associated with significant muscle hypertrophy, any strength training can help maintain metabolic rate, aiding in weight management.

Getting Started: Preparing for Bicep Curls
Before you dive into the bicep curl exercise, it's essential to ensure that you are physically ready and that you have the right equipment:

Consult with Your Doctor: Before starting any exercise program, it's a good idea to consult with your healthcare provider, especially if you have pre-existing health conditions or concerns.

Choose the Right Weights: For seniors, starting with light weights—typically 1 to 5 pounds—is advisable. Choose a weight that feels manageable but still provides a challenge by the last few repetitions.

Gather Your Equipment: You'll need:

A sturdy chair (if you prefer to sit)
Light dumbbells or water bottles
An exercise mat (if standing)
Warm-Up: Always start with a gentle warm-up to prepare your muscles and joints. Simple movements like arm circles, shoulder rolls, and wrist rotations can help loosen up your upper body.

Step-by-Step Guide to Performing Bicep Curls
Now, let's get into the nitty-gritty of performing bicep curls correctly. Here's how to do it:

1. Starting Position:

Seated Position: Sit in a chair with your feet flat on the ground, hip-width apart. Allow your arms to hang naturally at your sides with a dumbbell in each hand, palms facing forward.
Standing Position: Stand with your feet shoulder-width apart, holding a dumbbell in each hand, arms fully extended at your sides, palms facing forward.

2. The Curl Movement:

Engage Your Core: Whether seated or standing, tighten your abdominal muscles to provide stability throughout the movement.
Lift the Weights: Slowly bend your elbows to lift the weights towards your shoulders. Keep your upper arms stationary and close to your torso; only your forearms should move.
Squeeze at the Top: When the weights reach shoulder height, pause for a moment and squeeze your biceps. This contraction maximizes muscle engagement.

3. Lowering the Weights:

Controlled Descent: Slowly lower the weights back to the starting position, fully extending your arms. It's essential to control the movement and avoid letting the weights drop quickly.
4. Repeat: Aim for 8 to 12 repetitions for one set. Rest for 30-60 seconds between sets. Start with 1-2 sets and gradually increase as you build strength.

Key Tips for Proper Form and Safety
Posture Matters: Maintain a straight back and avoid leaning forward or backward. Proper posture ensures you target the right muscles and reduces the risk of strain.
Don't Rush: Slow, controlled movements are more effective and safer than quick, jerky motions. Focus on the muscle engagement throughout the entire range of motion.

Listen to Your Body: If you feel any sharp pain or discomfort, stop immediately. It's crucial to differentiate between muscle fatigue and pain.

Incorporate Breathing: Exhale as you lift the weights and inhale as you lower them. Proper breathing can enhance performance and help you stay relaxed.

Consistency is Key: Aim to include bicep curls in your routine 2-3 times a week, allowing your muscles to rest in between sessions.

Modifications for Different Fitness Levels

If Standing is Difficult: Perform the curls while seated to minimize strain on your legs and lower back.

For Extra Support: Use a wall or the back of a chair for balance if you are standing and feel unsteady.

Increase Weight Gradually: As you become stronger, consider increasing the weight by small increments (0.5 to 1 pound) to continue challenging your muscles.

Resistance Bands: If weights become too easy, consider using resistance bands. They provide constant tension throughout the movement and can be adjusted based on your strength level.

Incorporating Bicep Curls into Your Fitness Routine

To reap the full benefits of bicep curls, integrate them into a balanced workout routine that includes:

Cardiovascular Exercise: Aim for at least 150 minutes of moderate-intensity aerobic activity weekly, such as walking, cycling, or swimming.

Flexibility and Stretching: Include stretching exercises, like the arm and shoulder stretches, to maintain flexibility and prevent tightness.

Other Strength Exercises: Complement your bicep curls with tricep exercises, shoulder presses, and seated rows to create a balanced upper-body strength program.

Bicep curls with light weights are a fantastic exercise for seniors looking to enhance their strength, improve functional fitness, and promote independence in daily activities. With proper technique, modifications, and a commitment to consistency, you can reap the rewards of this simple yet effective exercise. Remember, every little effort counts—celebrate your progress, no matter how small, and enjoy the journey to better health and well-being!

By incorporating bicep curls into your routine, you're taking a significant step towards a healthier, stronger you, so grab those weights and let's get started!

Overhead Press from the Chair

The overhead press is a fundamental exercise that can be tailored to suit individuals of all fitness levels, particularly seniors looking to maintain or improve their upper body strength. This seated version, often referred to as the "overhead press from the chair," is a safe and effective way to work on your shoulder, arm, and upper back muscles without the need to stand. For those over 60, this exercise not only helps build strength but also enhances overall stability, balance, and mobility, which are crucial for daily activities.

Benefits of the Overhead Press from the Chair
Improves Upper Body Strength: The overhead press primarily targets the deltoid muscles in the shoulders, along with the triceps and upper chest. This helps in lifting objects overhead safely, whether it's a grocery bag or a suitcase.

Enhances Stability and Balance: Seated exercises reduce the risk of falls and injuries, making them ideal for seniors. Strengthening the upper body improves your ability to perform daily tasks with more confidence.

Increases Range of Motion: Regularly performing this exercise can improve flexibility in the shoulder joints, making it easier to reach for items above your head.

Supports Posture: A strong upper body contributes to better posture, which is essential for preventing back and neck pain, particularly as we age.

Accessible and Convenient: You can do the overhead press from a stable chair at home, making it a convenient option for integrating strength training into your daily routine.

Getting Started: Preparation
Before you begin, ensure you have a sturdy chair without wheels and that your environment is free of obstacles. You will also need:

Dumbbells or Resistance Bands: Light weights (1-5 pounds) are ideal for beginners. If you don't have weights, resistance bands can provide an excellent alternative.

Comfortable Clothing: Wear fitted clothing that allows for a full range of motion but isn't too loose to avoid getting caught on anything.

Water Bottle: Stay hydrated before, during, and after your workout.

Steps to Perform the Overhead Press from the Chair

1. Setting Up

Sit Properly: Begin by sitting up straight in your chair with your feet flat on the ground. Position your knees directly above your ankles to maintain a stable base.

Engage Your Core: Sit tall, engaging your abdominal muscles. This will help support your spine during the movement.

Hold the Weights: Grab a dumbbell in each hand, or grasp the handles of your resistance band. If using weights, hold them at shoulder height with your palms facing forward. If using a band, step on the middle of the band with both feet and hold the handles at shoulder height.

2. Executing the Press

Press Upward: Slowly raise the weights overhead, extending your arms fully. Ensure your elbows are slightly forward (not locked out) and that your wrists are straight. Your movement should be controlled, not rushed.

Focus on Breathing: Inhale as you prepare to lift and exhale as you press the weights overhead. This rhythmic breathing will help you maintain stability and control.

Hold at the Top: At the peak of the movement, pause for a moment. This is crucial as it allows your muscles to engage fully. Imagine pushing the weights up through the ceiling; this visualization can enhance your focus.

3. Lowering the Weights

Return to Start Position: Slowly lower the weights back to shoulder height while inhaling. Ensure you maintain control during this phase; do not let the weights drop quickly.

Keep Your Core Engaged: Maintain your core engagement throughout the entire movement, both during the press and the return.

4. Repetitions and Sets

Start Slow: Aim for 8-12 repetitions for your first set. Rest for about 30 seconds before performing 2-3 additional sets, depending on your comfort and energy levels.

Progress Gradually: If you feel comfortable, gradually increase the weight or resistance as you gain strength. It's crucial to listen to your body and not push beyond your limits.

Tips for Proper Form

Maintain a Neutral Spine: Keep your back straight and avoid leaning forward or backward. If you find yourself leaning, reassess your seating position or the height of your weights.

Avoid Overextending: When pressing overhead, do not arch your back or raise your shoulders towards your ears. Instead, focus on keeping your shoulders relaxed and down.

Keep Elbows Slightly Forward: This positioning helps protect your shoulder joints during the exercise.

Modifications for Comfort
Lighter Weights: If you are new to strength training or feel any discomfort, start with lighter weights or resistance bands.

Range of Motion: If lifting weights overhead is uncomfortable, you can limit the range of motion by only raising the weights to shoulder height.

No Weights: If using weights is not an option, perform the exercise without them, focusing on the motion to build strength gradually.

Common Mistakes to Avoid
Rushing the Movement: Always maintain a controlled pace. Quick movements can lead to injury, especially in older adults.

Inadequate Warm-Up: Before starting any strength training routine, including the overhead press, ensure you perform a gentle warm-up to prepare your muscles and joints.

Ignoring Pain Signals: If you experience pain (not just discomfort) during the exercise, stop immediately and consult a healthcare professional if necessary.

Incorporating the overhead press from the chair into your regular exercise routine can significantly enhance your upper body strength, flexibility, and overall quality of life. Remember, consistency is key. Aim to practice this exercise 2-3 times a week, and you'll soon notice improvements in your ability to perform daily activities with greater ease and confidence.

Always consult with a healthcare provider before beginning any new exercise program, especially if you have pre-existing conditions or concerns. Enjoy your journey towards improved fitness and well-being!

Seated Side Leg Raises

Seated Side Leg Raises are a fantastic exercise for seniors, especially those looking to improve their strength, flexibility, and overall mobility. This exercise focuses primarily on the hip abductors—the muscles located on the outside of your hips and thighs. Strengthening these muscles is crucial for maintaining balance, stability, and independence in daily activities. In this guide, we'll delve into the benefits, proper technique, variations, and tips for incorporating Seated Side Leg Raises into your fitness routine.

Understanding the Exercise
What Are Seated Side Leg Raises?

Seated Side Leg Raises involve lifting one leg to the side while sitting in a chair. This movement primarily targets the gluteus medius and minimus, which are essential for hip stability. The exercise is simple yet effective, making it accessible for seniors, beginners, or those recovering from injury.

Benefits of Seated Side Leg Raises
Strengthens Hip Muscles
By engaging the hip abductors, this exercise helps build strength in the outer thighs and hips, which is vital for walking, climbing stairs, and performing daily activities.

Improves Balance and Stability
Strong hip muscles contribute significantly to balance. Improved stability helps reduce the risk of falls—a common concern for seniors.

Enhances Flexibility
Regular practice of Seated Side Leg Raises can increase flexibility in the hips and thighs, allowing for a greater range of motion in daily movements.

Promotes Joint Health
Strengthening the muscles around the hips can help support the hip joint, potentially reducing the risk of joint-related issues like arthritis.

Easy to Perform
This exercise can be done in the comfort of your home, making it easy to integrate into your daily routine without requiring any special equipment.

How to Perform Seated Side Leg Raises
Preparation

Choose the Right Chair: Select a sturdy chair without arms that allows you to sit comfortably with your feet flat on the floor. Ensure it is stable and won't slide around during the exercise.

Dress Comfortably: Wear loose-fitting clothing that allows for easy movement. Avoid tight pants that might restrict your range of motion.

Warm-Up: Before performing the exercise, engage in a brief warm-up. This could include light marching in place, shoulder rolls, or gentle neck stretches to prepare your body for movement.

Step-by-Step Instructions

Sit Up Straight: Begin by sitting at the edge of the chair with your back straight and shoulders relaxed. Your feet should be flat on the floor, hip-width apart. Engage your core muscles to stabilize your torso.

Position Your Legs: Keep your right leg extended in front of you, with your knee slightly bent. Your left leg will be the one you raise.

Lift the Left Leg: Slowly raise your left leg out to the side. Keep your foot flexed (toes pointing straight ahead) and your knee slightly bent. Lift your leg until it is parallel to the ground or as high as you can comfortably go without straining.

Hold the Position: Pause for a moment at the top of the lift, feeling the contraction in your hip and thigh muscles. Hold for 1-2 seconds.

Lower the Leg: Gradually lower your left leg back to the starting position. Focus on a controlled movement to avoid any sudden jerks.

Repeat: Perform 10-15 repetitions on the left side, then switch to the right leg and repeat the same number of repetitions.

Rest and Repeat: After completing one set on each side, rest for 30 seconds to a minute before repeating for a total of 2-3 sets.

Tips for Success
Focus on Form: Maintaining proper form is essential for maximizing benefits and preventing injury. Keep your back straight and avoid leaning to one side as you lift your leg.

Breathe: Remember to breathe throughout the exercise. Inhale as you lower your leg and exhale as you lift it.

Use Resistance Bands: For added difficulty, consider using resistance bands around your thighs to increase the intensity of the exercise. This can enhance muscle engagement and promote strength gains.

Modify as Needed: If lifting your leg to the side is too challenging, you can start with smaller movements and gradually increase the height of your leg as you gain strength and confidence.

Incorporate Variations: To keep your routine interesting, mix in variations such as lifting your leg straight out in front of you or adding ankle weights once you feel comfortable with the basic movement.

Common Mistakes to Avoid
Leaning Back: Ensure your torso remains upright throughout the exercise. Leaning back can put unnecessary strain on your lower back and reduce the effectiveness of the movement.

Using Momentum: Avoid swinging your leg up using momentum. Focus on controlled movements to engage the correct muscles and minimize the risk of injury.

Overextending: Don't lift your leg higher than your comfort level. It's essential to listen to your body and respect your range of motion.

Seated Side Leg Raises are a simple yet powerful exercise that can contribute significantly to your strength, flexibility, and overall well-being. By incorporating this exercise into your routine, you are taking an essential step towards maintaining your independence and enhancing your quality of life as you age. Remember to stay consistent, listen to your body, and enjoy the journey to greater mobility and strength. As with any exercise program, consult with a healthcare professional before starting, especially if you have any existing health conditions or concerns.

Embrace this exercise, and make it a regular part of your fitness regimen. Over time, you'll likely notice improvements in your balance, strength, and daily function, helping you to stay active and engaged in life well into your senior years.

Creating a Simple Strength Routine for Muscle Maintenance

As we age, maintaining muscle mass and strength becomes increasingly important for our overall health and functional independence. For seniors, especially those over 60, a simple strength routine can significantly enhance mobility, balance, and quality of life. This chapter will guide you through creating an effective strength training regimen tailored to your needs, using safe and accessible exercises.

Why Muscle Maintenance Matters
Muscle maintenance is essential for several reasons:

Functional Independence: Strong muscles support daily activities such as climbing stairs, lifting objects, and getting up from a chair. This independence enhances self-esteem and reduces the risk of falls.

Metabolic Health: Muscle tissue is metabolically active, meaning that it helps burn calories even at rest. Maintaining muscle mass can aid in weight management and improve insulin sensitivity, which is crucial for preventing type 2 diabetes.

Joint Support: Strong muscles around joints provide stability and reduce the risk of injuries. This is particularly important as we age and our ligaments and tendons become less resilient.

Bone Health: Strength training can improve bone density, which is vital for preventing osteoporosis and fractures.

Mental Well-Being: Engaging in regular physical activity releases endorphins, which can enhance mood and decrease feelings of anxiety and depression.

Assessing Your Fitness Level
Before starting any new exercise routine, it's essential to assess your current fitness level. Here are some considerations:

Consult a Healthcare Professional: Always check with your doctor, especially if you have chronic health conditions or have been inactive.

Self-Assessment: Consider your ability to perform daily tasks. Can you lift groceries, get up from a seated position, or climb stairs without difficulty? This will help you identify your starting point.

Basic Equipment for Strength Training
For a simple strength routine, you'll need minimal equipment. Here are some essentials:

Light Dumbbells: Start with weights that you can lift comfortably for 10-15 repetitions. For many seniors, 1-5 pounds is sufficient.

Resistance Bands: These versatile bands come in various resistance levels and can be used for many exercises. They are portable and easy to store.

Sturdy Chair: A firm, stable chair is crucial for seated exercises and support during standing exercises.

Exercise Mat: If you're doing floor exercises or stretches, a comfortable mat can provide cushioning.

Designing Your Strength Routine
Frequency: Aim for at least two days of strength training per week, allowing for rest days in between. Consistency is key to building strength.

Structure: A well-rounded strength routine includes exercises for all major muscle groups: upper body, lower body, and core. Here's a sample structure for your routine:

Warm-Up (5-10 Minutes): Begin with light activities like marching in place, shoulder rolls, or gentle stretching. This helps prepare your muscles and joints for exercise and reduces the risk of injury.

Upper Body Exercises:

Seated Dumbbell Press: Sit in a chair with a dumbbell in each hand. Start with your arms at shoulder height, palms facing forward. Press the weights overhead until your arms are fully extended, then lower them back to the starting position. Aim for 10-15 repetitions.

Bicep Curls: While seated or standing, hold a dumbbell in each hand with your arms at your sides, palms facing forward. Curl the weights toward your shoulders, keeping your elbows close to your body. Lower the weights slowly. Perform 10-15 repetitions.

Tricep Extensions: Sit or stand and hold one dumbbell with both hands above your head, arms extended. Lower the weight behind your head by bending your elbows, then return to the starting position. Aim for 10-15 repetitions.

Lower Body Exercises:

Chair Squats: Stand in front of a sturdy chair. Lower yourself as if you're going to sit down, but stop just above the chair and rise back up. This builds strength in the legs and glutes. Repeat for 10-15 repetitions.

Seated Leg Lifts: Sit in a chair with your back straight. Extend one leg straight out in front of you, keeping it parallel to the ground. Hold for a few seconds, then lower it back down. Switch legs and repeat for 10-15 repetitions on each side.

Calf Raises: Stand behind your chair for support. Raise your heels off the ground, standing on your toes, then lower back down. Repeat for 10-15 repetitions.

Core Exercises:

Seated Marching: Sit tall in a chair and lift your knees alternately as if marching in place. This engages your core and improves balance. Aim for 10-15 repetitions on each side.

Torso Twists: Sit in a chair and place your hands on your shoulders. Twist your upper body to the right, then to the left, keeping your hips stable. Repeat for 10-15 repetitions.

Chair Leg Extensions: While seated, extend one leg straight out and hold for a few seconds. Alternate legs for a total of 10-15 repetitions.

Cool Down (5-10 Minutes): Finish your routine with gentle stretches for all major muscle groups. Focus on breathing deeply to lower your heart rate and relax your muscles.

Modifications and Progression
It's essential to listen to your body and make modifications as needed. If an exercise feels too challenging, reduce the weight, decrease the number of repetitions, or perform the exercise seated instead of standing. As you gain strength and confidence, gradually increase the weight, the number of repetitions, or the difficulty of the exercises.

Safety Tips
Listen to Your Body: If you feel pain (beyond normal muscle fatigue), stop the exercise immediately. Consult a professional if you experience persistent discomfort.

Maintain Proper Form: Focus on your technique to avoid injury. Keep movements controlled and avoid jerking or bouncing.

Stay Hydrated: Drink water before, during, and after your workout to keep your body hydrated.

Use Support as Needed: Use a chair or wall for balance during standing exercises, especially if you're feeling unsteady.

Creating a simple strength routine tailored for muscle maintenance doesn't have to be complicated. By focusing on consistency, proper form, and gradual progression, you can build strength and improve your overall well-being. Remember, the goal is to enhance your quality of life, enabling you to perform daily activities with ease and confidence. Embrace the journey, and celebrate every achievement, no matter how small. Your body will thank you for it!

Chapter 5: Stretching for Flexibility and Pain Relief

Importance of Stretching for Seniors

As we age, maintaining flexibility becomes essential for overall health and well-being. Stretching is not just an afterthought in a workout routine; it is a crucial component of a balanced exercise program, especially for seniors. Here, we will explore the various benefits of stretching, how it impacts your body, and practical tips for incorporating stretching into your daily life.

Understanding Flexibility and Its Decline with Age
Flexibility refers to the range of motion in your joints and muscles. It is an important aspect of physical fitness that often declines with age due to factors such as sedentary lifestyles, muscle stiffness, and joint degeneration. As we age, our muscles and connective tissues become less elastic, leading to stiffness and reduced mobility. This loss of flexibility can affect our ability to perform daily activities, increase the risk of falls, and contribute to chronic pain conditions.

Research indicates that after the age of 40, we lose about 1% of muscle mass and strength each year. This decline can be accelerated by inactivity and can lead to a vicious cycle: decreased flexibility makes exercise more difficult, leading to further inactivity and reduced flexibility. Stretching can play a pivotal role in breaking this cycle.

Benefits of Stretching for Seniors
Enhanced Mobility and Flexibility:
Regular stretching helps to maintain and improve flexibility, which is vital for performing everyday tasks such as bending, reaching, and turning. Improved flexibility allows seniors to move more freely and confidently, which can enhance their quality of life.

Injury Prevention:
As flexibility declines, the risk of injuries—such as strains and sprains—can increase. Stretching prepares the muscles and joints for physical activity, reducing the risk of injury. It warms up the muscles, making them less prone to damage during exercise or daily movements.

Improved Posture:
Good posture is critical for overall body alignment and health. Stretching strengthens the muscles responsible for maintaining proper posture while loosening tight muscles that can pull the body out of alignment. This is particularly important for seniors, as poor posture can lead to back pain and other issues.

Enhanced Blood Circulation:
Stretching promotes better blood circulation throughout the body. Improved circulation helps deliver oxygen and nutrients to muscles and organs, supporting overall health and recovery. Better circulation can also aid in reducing muscle soreness and stiffness.

Stress Relief and Relaxation:
Stretching is not just physical; it also has mental benefits. The act of stretching encourages relaxation, reduces stress, and promotes a sense of well-being. Incorporating deep breathing into your stretching routine can further enhance these benefits, calming the mind and body.

Alleviation of Muscle Tension and Pain:
Many seniors experience muscle tension and pain, particularly in the back, neck, and shoulders. Regular stretching can help relieve this tension, reducing discomfort and enhancing overall mobility. It can be particularly beneficial for those with conditions such as arthritis, as gentle stretching can alleviate stiffness in the joints.

Improved Balance and Coordination:
Stretching can help improve balance and coordination, both of which are crucial for preventing falls—a significant risk for seniors. Stretching exercises that focus on the lower body, such as hamstring and calf stretches, can particularly benefit balance.

Support for Mental Health:
Engaging in regular stretching can promote a positive mood and reduce symptoms of anxiety and depression. The mindful aspect of stretching encourages a connection between body and mind, fostering a sense of calm and control over one's physical well-being.

Practical Stretching Tips for Seniors
While the benefits of stretching are clear, it's important to approach stretching with care and intention. Here are some practical tips for seniors to incorporate stretching into their daily routines safely and effectively:

Warm Up First:
Before stretching, it's crucial to warm up your muscles with light aerobic activity. This could include a short walk or gentle movement to get the blood flowing and prepare your body for stretching.

Focus on Major Muscle Groups:
Target the major muscle groups, including the neck, shoulders, back, hips, legs, and ankles. Ensure that you stretch both sides of the body evenly.

Hold Each Stretch:
When stretching, hold each position for at least 15-30 seconds. This duration allows the muscles to relax and elongate effectively. Avoid bouncing during stretches, as this can lead to injury.

Listen to Your Body:
Stretching should feel good, not painful. Pay attention to your body's signals and ease into each stretch. If you feel pain, back off the stretch slightly.

Be Consistent:
Incorporate stretching into your routine at least 2-3 times per week. Daily stretching is even better, as it can lead to gradual improvements in flexibility and mobility over time.

Use Props When Necessary:
Chairs, straps, or even towels can assist in achieving a good stretch without straining. For seniors, using a sturdy chair for seated stretches can provide support and stability.

Try Guided Sessions:
Participating in a class or following a video led by a certified instructor can be helpful, especially for beginners. Look for classes specifically designed for seniors, as they will be tailored to your needs.

Include Breathing Techniques:
Incorporate deep breathing into your stretching routine. Inhale as you prepare to stretch and exhale as you deepen the stretch. This practice enhances relaxation and oxygen flow.

Sample Stretching Routine for Seniors
To get started, here's a simple stretching routine tailored for seniors:

Neck Stretch:

Sit comfortably in a chair.
Slowly tilt your head to one side, bringing your ear toward your shoulder. Hold for 15-30 seconds. Repeat on the other side.
Shoulder Rolls:

Sit or stand with arms relaxed at your sides.
Roll your shoulders forward in a circular motion, then reverse the direction. Repeat 5-10 times.
Seated Hamstring Stretch:

While seated, extend one leg straight in front of you with the heel on the floor.

Keep the other foot flat on the ground.
Gently lean forward toward your extended leg, feeling a stretch in the back of your thigh. Hold for 15-30 seconds, then switch legs.
Cat-Cow Stretch:

Sit at the edge of your chair.
Inhale as you arch your back (Cow), and exhale as you round your spine (Cat). Repeat 5-10 times.
Seated Forward Bend:

While seated, extend your arms overhead.
Exhale as you bend forward from your hips, reaching for your toes. Hold for 15-30 seconds.
Ankle Rolls:

While seated, lift one foot off the ground.
Roll your ankle in a circular motion, then switch directions. Repeat for 5-10 rolls on each ankle.

Stretching is a vital practice that offers numerous benefits for seniors, from improved flexibility and mobility to enhanced mental well-being. By incorporating regular stretching into your daily routine, you can maintain your independence, enhance your quality of life, and reduce the risk of injury as you age. Remember, the goal of stretching is not only to feel better physically but also to enjoy the process and connect with your body in a meaningful way. So, take a moment each day to stretch, breathe, and embrace the vitality that comes with movement.

The Best Stretches for Mobility and Joint Health

As we age, maintaining mobility and joint health becomes increasingly important for our overall well-being and quality of life. Regular stretching can help enhance flexibility, reduce stiffness, prevent injury, and improve posture. Here, we'll delve into the best stretches that cater specifically to enhancing mobility and promoting joint health, ensuring you remain active and comfortable in your daily life.

Understanding Mobility and Joint Health
Mobility refers to the ability to move freely and easily, which is essential for performing daily activities. Joint health, on the other hand, involves maintaining the integrity and functionality of the joints, which serve as the connections between bones. Good joint health allows for smoother movement and less pain. Incorporating stretching into your routine can significantly contribute to both mobility and joint health by:

Increasing flexibility: Stretching helps lengthen muscles and improve the range of motion around the joints.

Reducing stiffness: Regular stretching can alleviate stiffness that often accompanies aging or prolonged periods of inactivity.

Enhancing blood circulation: Stretching promotes blood flow to muscles and joints, which can aid in recovery and reduce soreness.

Preventing injuries: Flexible muscles are less likely to be strained or pulled during physical activity.

Improving posture: Stretching can correct muscle imbalances and promote proper alignment, reducing strain on the joints.

Key Stretches for Enhanced Mobility and Joint Health

Here are some of the most effective stretches that focus on different areas of the body. Each stretch should be performed gently, and you should never force your body into a position that causes pain. Hold each stretch for about 15 to 30 seconds, breathing deeply and relaxing into the stretch.

1. Neck Stretch

Purpose: Alleviates tension in the neck and improves cervical mobility.

How to Do It:
Sit or stand up straight with your shoulders relaxed.
Slowly tilt your head to one side, bringing your ear toward your shoulder.
To deepen the stretch, you can gently place your hand on the opposite side of your head.
Hold for 15-30 seconds, then switch sides.

2. Shoulder Rolls

Purpose: Relieves tension in the shoulders and upper back.

How to Do It:
Stand or sit comfortably with your arms at your sides.
Inhale as you lift your shoulders toward your ears.
Exhale as you roll your shoulders back and down.
Repeat for 5-10 rolls, then switch directions.

3. Chest Stretch

Purpose: Opens up the chest and improves shoulder mobility.

How to Do It:
Stand in a doorway with your arms raised at shoulder height, elbows bent.
Place your forearms against the door frame.
Lean slightly forward until you feel a stretch in your chest.
Hold for 15-30 seconds.

4. Upper Back Stretch
Purpose: Enhances flexibility in the upper back and shoulders.

How to Do It:
Sit or stand tall.
Interlace your fingers and extend your arms forward, rounding your upper back.
Tuck your chin to your chest and feel the stretch across your upper back.
Hold for 15-30 seconds.

5. Torso Twist
Purpose: Increases spinal mobility and stretches the lower back.

How to Do It:
Sit in a chair with your feet flat on the ground.
Place your right hand on the back of the chair and twist your torso to the right.
Use your left hand on your right knee for support.
Hold for 15-30 seconds, then switch sides.

6. Seated Forward Bend
Purpose: Stretches the hamstrings and lower back.

How to Do It:
Sit on the floor with your legs extended in front of you.
Inhale as you raise your arms overhead.
Exhale and hinge at your hips to reach forward toward your toes.
Keep your back straight and hold for 15-30 seconds.

7. Hip Flexor Stretch
Purpose: Relieves tightness in the hips and improves hip mobility.

How to Do It:
Start in a lunge position with your right foot forward and left knee on the ground.
Shift your weight forward until you feel a stretch in the front of your left hip.
Keep your back straight and hold for 15-30 seconds, then switch sides.

8. Quadriceps Stretch
Purpose: Increases flexibility in the front of the thigh.

How to Do It:
Stand with your feet hip-width apart.
Bend your right knee and bring your heel toward your glutes.
Hold your ankle with your right hand and keep your knees together.
Hold for 15-30 seconds, then switch sides.

9. Calf Stretch

Purpose: Improves ankle flexibility and stretches the calf muscles.

How to Do It:
Stand facing a wall with your hands pressed against it.
Step your right foot back, keeping it straight and your left knee bent.
Lean into the wall until you feel a stretch in your right calf.
Hold for 15-30 seconds, then switch sides.

10. Seated Figure Four Stretch

Purpose: Opens the hips and stretches the outer thighs.

How to Do It:
Sit on a chair and place your right ankle over your left knee.
Gently press down on your right knee and lean forward slightly.
Hold for 15-30 seconds, then switch sides.

Tips for Effective Stretching

Warm Up First: It's beneficial to warm up your body with light activity (like walking) for 5-10 minutes before stretching.

Breathe Deeply: Focus on your breath. Inhale deeply through your nose, and exhale slowly through your mouth. This can help you relax into the stretches.

Listen to Your Body: Stretch only to the point of mild discomfort, not pain. If a stretch feels painful, ease off until you find a comfortable position.

Be Consistent: Incorporate these stretches into your daily routine. Aim for at least 3-4 times a week to see significant benefits.

Stay Hydrated: Proper hydration is vital for joint health and can help keep your muscles supple.

Incorporating these stretches into your routine will not only enhance your mobility but also promote overall joint health. Regular stretching can lead to increased flexibility, reduced risk of injury, and an overall better quality of life. Remember to be patient and consistent, and soon you'll notice improvements in your mobility, comfort, and confidence in your movements. Always consult with a healthcare professional before beginning any new exercise regimen, especially if you have existing health concerns or conditions. Embrace the journey to better mobility, and enjoy the freedom it brings!

Neck Stretch

As we age, maintaining flexibility and mobility in our bodies becomes increasingly important. One area that often suffers from tension and tightness is the neck. For seniors, a well-executed neck stretch can provide significant relief from discomfort, enhance mobility, and contribute to overall well-being. In this detailed guide, we'll explore the anatomy of the neck, the benefits of neck stretching, a step-by-step stretching routine, and some helpful tips for ensuring that your stretching practice is both safe and effective.

Understanding the Neck: Anatomy and Importance
The neck, or cervical spine, consists of seven vertebrae (C1-C7) and supports the head while allowing for a wide range of motion. This area contains several muscles, ligaments, and nerves that work together to facilitate movement and support. Some of the key muscles involved in neck movement include:

Sternocleidomastoid: This muscle runs from the back of the skull to the collarbone and plays a critical role in turning and tilting the head.
Trapezius: This large muscle extends from the back of the neck down to the middle of the back and across to the shoulders, helping to lift and rotate the shoulder blades.
Levator Scapulae: Located at the back and side of the neck, this muscle elevates the shoulder blade and aids in neck movement.
The Importance of Neck Stretches
Relieving Tension and Pain: As we age, it's common to experience stiffness or discomfort in the neck due to poor posture, sedentary lifestyles, or stress. Regular stretching can alleviate this tension, helping to reduce pain and discomfort.

Improving Range of Motion: Incorporating neck stretches into your routine enhances flexibility and mobility. This is particularly beneficial for seniors who may find everyday tasks, such as looking over their shoulder while driving, increasingly difficult.

Promoting Better Posture: Stretching helps to counteract the effects of poor posture, especially for those who spend extended periods sitting or working at a computer. Improved posture not only feels better but can also contribute to better breathing and circulation.

Enhancing Blood Flow: Stretching increases blood circulation to the muscles and surrounding tissues, promoting healing and reducing recovery time from minor injuries.

Reducing Headaches: Tightness in the neck can contribute to tension headaches. Regular stretching can alleviate this tightness, potentially reducing the frequency and severity of headaches.

Step-by-Step Neck Stretching Routine

Before beginning any stretching routine, it's essential to warm up the body gently to prepare the muscles. You can do this by moving your shoulders in circular motions, taking deep breaths, and gently rolling your head from side to side.

1. Neck Side Stretch

How to Perform:

Sit or stand comfortably with your back straight.
Keep your shoulders relaxed and down.
Slowly tilt your head to the right, bringing your ear toward your shoulder.
You can gently place your right hand on the left side of your head to deepen the stretch (but do not pull).
Hold this position for 15-30 seconds, breathing deeply and feeling the stretch along the left side of your neck.
Return to the center and repeat on the left side.
Tips:

Avoid raising your shoulder towards your ear; focus on bringing the ear closer to the shoulder.
If you feel any sharp pain, ease out of the stretch.

2. Neck Forward Stretch

How to Perform:

Sit upright in a chair or stand with your feet shoulder-width apart.
Interlace your fingers and place your hands on the back of your head.
Gently press down with your hands, bringing your chin toward your chest.
Hold this position for 15-30 seconds, feeling the stretch along the back of your neck and upper back.
Tips:

Keep your shoulders relaxed and avoid slumping; maintain a straight back.
If you experience discomfort, ease off the pressure.

3. Neck Rotation Stretch

How to Perform:

Begin in a seated or standing position with your back straight.
Turn your head to the right, aiming to look over your shoulder.
Hold this position for 15-30 seconds, feeling the stretch along the left side of your neck.
Slowly return to the center and repeat on the left side.

Tips:

Keep your movements slow and controlled; avoid jerking or rushing through the stretch.
Make sure to keep your shoulders level and relaxed throughout the movement.

4. Chin Tuck Stretch

How to Perform:

Sit or stand tall with your shoulders relaxed.
Gently tuck your chin toward your chest, keeping your back straight.
Hold for 5-10 seconds and then release.
Repeat this 5-10 times to help strengthen the muscles in your neck and improve posture.

Tips:

Focus on a smooth motion; do not force the movement.
This stretch can be done throughout the day, especially if you spend long hours at a computer.

Best Practices for Neck Stretching

Warm Up: Always warm up your muscles before stretching to prevent injury. A few minutes of light aerobic activity, such as walking, can help.

Listen to Your Body: Pay attention to how your neck feels during stretches. If you experience sharp pain or discomfort, stop the exercise.

Breathe Deeply: Focus on your breath. Inhale deeply as you prepare to stretch, and exhale slowly as you move into the stretch. This helps relax the muscles and can enhance the effectiveness of the stretch.

Consistency is Key: Aim to incorporate neck stretches into your daily routine. Just a few minutes each day can lead to significant improvements in flexibility and reduced discomfort.

Seek Professional Guidance: If you're unsure about your form or experience chronic pain, consider consulting a physical therapist or fitness professional. They can provide tailored advice and ensure you're performing stretches correctly.

Neck stretches are a vital part of maintaining overall health and well-being, especially for seniors over 60. They help alleviate tension, improve flexibility, and promote better posture, all of which contribute to a better quality of life. By integrating these stretches into your daily routine, you can experience the benefits of a more flexible and pain-free neck. Remember, consistency is crucial, and listening to your body is essential for a safe and effective stretching practice.

Shoulder and Arm Stretch

Among the various parts of our body, the shoulders and arms are pivotal in almost every movement we make, whether lifting a grocery bag, reaching for something on a high shelf, or even sitting at a desk. Regular stretching can help alleviate tension, enhance flexibility, and prevent injuries. In this section, we will explore the importance of shoulder and arm stretches, the anatomy involved, step-by-step instructions for effective stretches, and some helpful tips to integrate them into your daily routine.

Why Stretching Your Shoulders and Arms is Important
Improved Flexibility: Stretching helps maintain and improve the range of motion in your shoulders and arms. As we age, our muscles and joints tend to become stiffer, making everyday tasks more challenging. Regular stretching counteracts this stiffness.

Injury Prevention: By increasing flexibility, you reduce the risk of injuries related to overexertion or sudden movements. Stretching helps to warm up your muscles, making them less prone to strains and tears.

Relief from Pain and Discomfort: Many seniors experience discomfort in their shoulders and arms due to arthritis, bursitis, or tendinitis. Gentle stretches can alleviate tightness and pain, promoting better overall mobility.

Enhanced Posture: Poor posture can lead to shoulder and arm tension. Regular stretching helps to open up tight areas and encourage better alignment, reducing strain on your muscles and joints.

Better Circulation: Stretching increases blood flow to the muscles, enhancing circulation. This can help with recovery from soreness and improve overall vitality.

Mind-Body Connection: Stretching is also an excellent way to connect your mind and body, promoting relaxation and mindfulness. It encourages deep breathing and awareness of your physical state, which can be beneficial for mental health.

Anatomy of the Shoulder and Arm
Before we dive into the stretches, it's helpful to understand the anatomy of the shoulder and arm. The shoulder is a complex joint formed by the upper arm bone (humerus), shoulder blade (scapula), and collarbone (clavicle). Key muscles involved in shoulder and arm movement include:

Deltoids: The primary muscles covering the shoulder, responsible for lifting the arm.

Rotator Cuff Muscles: A group of four muscles that stabilize the shoulder joint and allow for a wide range of movement.

Biceps Brachii: Located in the upper arm, these muscles are crucial for lifting and pulling motions.

Triceps Brachii: Located on the back of the upper arm, they are essential for extending the elbow.

Step-by-Step Instructions for Shoulder and Arm Stretches

1. Seated Shoulder Stretch

Benefits: This stretch targets the deltoids and helps relieve tension in the shoulder area.

Instructions:

Sit comfortably in a sturdy chair with your feet flat on the floor and your back straight.
Take a deep breath in, lifting both arms overhead.
As you exhale, lower your right arm and bring your left arm across your body.
Use your right hand to gently pull your left arm closer to your chest.
Hold this position for 15 to 30 seconds, feeling the stretch across your shoulder.
Repeat on the opposite side, bringing your right arm across your body and using your left hand to pull it gently.

2. Cross-Body Arm Stretch

Benefits: This stretch is effective for the shoulders and upper back, promoting overall flexibility.

Instructions:

Stand or sit with your back straight and feet shoulder-width apart.
Extend your right arm straight across your body at shoulder height.
With your left hand, gently pull your right arm towards your chest.
Keep your shoulder down and away from your ear to avoid tension.
Hold for 15 to 30 seconds, breathing deeply.
Switch sides, extending your left arm across your body and pulling gently with your right hand.

3. Overhead Tricep Stretch

Benefits: This stretch targets the triceps and shoulder area, improving flexibility and relieving tightness.

Instructions:

Stand or sit up straight.
Raise your right arm overhead, bending at the elbow so that your hand reaches down your back.
Use your left hand to gently push your right elbow back, deepening the stretch.
Hold this position for 15 to 30 seconds, feeling the stretch along your triceps and shoulders.
Switch arms and repeat.

4. Wall Angels
Benefits: This stretch helps open up the chest and shoulders, improving posture and flexibility.

Instructions:

Stand with your back against a wall, feet slightly away from the wall, and knees slightly bent.
Keep your lower back flat against the wall.
Raise both arms to shoulder height, elbows bent at 90 degrees, with the backs of your hands touching the wall.
Slowly slide your arms up the wall, maintaining contact with the wall, until they are fully extended.
Bring them back down to the starting position.
Repeat this movement 8-10 times, focusing on controlled movement and breathing.

5. Shoulder Rolls
Benefits: This dynamic stretch helps release tension and improve mobility in the shoulder joints.

Instructions:

Sit or stand comfortably with your arms at your sides.
Inhale as you lift your shoulders towards your ears.
Exhale as you roll your shoulders back and down, completing a full circular motion.
Perform 5-10 rolls in one direction, then switch and roll in the opposite direction.

Tips for Effective Stretching

Warm Up First: Always start with a gentle warm-up to increase blood flow to your muscles. This could include light walking or marching in place for a few minutes.

Breathe Deeply: Focus on your breath as you stretch. Inhale deeply through your nose and exhale slowly through your mouth. This can help relax your muscles and enhance the effectiveness of the stretch.

Listen to Your Body: Stretching should never be painful. If you feel any sharp pain, ease off the stretch. It's essential to respect your body's limits.

Consistency is Key: Aim to incorporate shoulder and arm stretches into your daily routine. Even a few minutes a day can lead to significant improvements in flexibility and comfort.

Use Props if Needed: If reaching or holding a stretch is challenging, consider using a strap, towel, or even a sturdy band to assist you.

Integrating Stretches into Your Routine

To maximize the benefits of these shoulder and arm stretches, consider integrating them into your daily activities. For example, you can perform these stretches in the morning as part of your wake-up routine or during breaks while watching TV. Setting aside a dedicated time for stretching, such as after a short walk or exercise session, can also enhance the overall experience.

Incorporating shoulder and arm stretches into your daily routine is an invaluable practice for maintaining flexibility, improving mobility, and preventing discomfort as you age. By focusing on gentle, effective stretches, you can enhance your overall well-being and enjoy a more active, fulfilling lifestyle. Remember that consistency is vital, so be patient with yourself as you work toward your flexibility and strength goals. With each stretch, you are investing in a healthier, more vibrant future.

Lower Back Stretch

Lower back pain is a common complaint among seniors, often stemming from a lack of flexibility, poor posture, or prolonged sitting. However, incorporating simple stretches into your daily routine can significantly alleviate discomfort, enhance mobility, and improve your overall quality of life. This chapter will delve deep into the lower back stretch, exploring its benefits, techniques, and tips for optimal results.

Understanding the Anatomy of the Lower Back
Before we dive into the stretches, it's essential to understand the anatomy of the lower back. The lower back, or lumbar region, consists of five vertebrae (L1-L5) supported by muscles, ligaments, and tendons. This area is crucial for supporting the upper body, allowing movement, and maintaining posture.

Common Causes of Lower Back Pain:

Muscle Strain: Often due to lifting heavy objects or sudden movements.
Herniated Discs: When the cushioning between the vertebrae bulges or ruptures.
Arthritis: Degenerative changes can lead to stiffness and pain.
Poor Posture: Sitting or standing incorrectly for long periods.
Sedentary Lifestyle: Lack of movement can weaken muscles and decrease flexibility.
The Importance of Lower Back Stretches
Incorporating lower back stretches into your routine can provide numerous benefits, including:

Increased Flexibility: Regular stretching helps lengthen muscles and tendons, improving overall flexibility in the lower back and hips.

Pain Relief: Stretching can relieve tension and tightness, reducing discomfort in the lower back.

Improved Posture: Strengthening and stretching the muscles in the lower back can promote better alignment, which is essential for reducing strain.

Enhanced Mobility: Stretching increases the range of motion, making everyday activities easier and more enjoyable.

Stress Reduction: Gentle stretching can also help calm the mind and reduce stress, which can contribute to muscle tension.

Preparing for Lower Back Stretches
Before starting any stretching routine, it's important to prepare your body. Here's how to get ready for your lower back stretches:

Find a Comfortable Space: Choose a quiet area where you can move freely without distractions. Use a mat or soft surface to sit or lie on.

Wear Comfortable Clothing: Opt for loose-fitting clothes that allow for movement. Avoid tight or restrictive garments.

Start with a Warm-Up: Spend a few minutes warming up your muscles. Simple activities like marching in place or gentle side bends can help increase blood flow and prepare your body for stretching.

Effective Lower Back Stretches
Here are several effective lower back stretches you can incorporate into your routine. Remember to listen to your body and never push yourself to the point of pain. Hold each stretch for 15-30 seconds and repeat 2-3 times.

1. Cat-Cow Stretch

The Cat-Cow stretch is a gentle way to mobilize the spine and relieve tension in the lower back.

How to Perform:

Begin on your hands and knees in a tabletop position, with your wrists aligned under your shoulders and knees under your hips.
Inhale as you arch your back, lifting your head and tailbone toward the ceiling (Cow).
Exhale as you round your back, tucking your chin to your chest and pulling your belly button toward your spine (Cat).

Repeat this sequence 5-10 times, moving slowly and synchronizing your breath with each movement.

2. Seated Forward Bend

This stretch targets the hamstrings and lower back, promoting flexibility and relaxation.

How to Perform:

Sit on the floor with your legs extended in front of you, keeping your back straight.
Inhale and reach your arms overhead, lengthening your spine.
Exhale as you hinge at your hips, reaching toward your toes. Keep your back straight and avoid rounding your shoulders.
If you can't reach your toes, rest your hands on your shins or thighs. Hold this position for 15-30 seconds, breathing deeply.

3. Knee-to-Chest Stretch

This stretch helps relieve lower back tension by gently stretching the lumbar region.

How to Perform:

Lie on your back with your knees bent and feet flat on the floor.
Slowly bring one knee toward your chest, using your hands to pull it closer.
Keep the opposite foot flat on the floor or extend it straight out for a deeper stretch.
Hold for 15-30 seconds, then switch legs. Repeat 2-3 times on each side.

4. Supine Spinal Twist

This stretch encourages spinal mobility and relieves tension in the lower back.

How to Perform:

Lie on your back with your knees bent and feet flat on the floor.
Extend your arms out to the sides, forming a T shape with your body.
Gently lower both knees to one side while keeping your shoulders on the floor.
Hold for 15-30 seconds, feeling the stretch in your lower back. Return to the starting position and repeat on the other side.

5. Child's Pose

Child's Pose is a restorative stretch that promotes relaxation and stretches the lower back.

How to Perform:

Start on your hands and knees in a tabletop position.

Sit back on your heels, reaching your arms forward and lowering your forehead to the floor.

Allow your hips to sink back and relax into the stretch. Hold for 30 seconds to a minute, breathing deeply and focusing on releasing tension in your lower back.

Tips for Effective Stretching

To get the most out of your lower back stretches, keep these tips in mind:

Breathe Deeply: Focus on your breath throughout each stretch. Inhale deeply to expand your chest and abdomen, and exhale slowly to relax into the stretch.

Stay Relaxed: Avoid tensing your muscles. Instead, allow your body to relax and sink into each stretch gently.

Listen to Your Body: Stretching should never be painful. If you feel sharp pain, ease off the stretch and consult a healthcare professional if necessary.

Be Consistent: Incorporate these stretches into your daily routine for the best results. Aim to stretch at least three to four times a week.

When to Consult a Professional

While stretching can be beneficial, it's essential to consult with a healthcare provider or physical therapist if you experience:

Persistent or severe lower back pain

Pain that radiates down your legs

Numbness or tingling sensations

Difficulty performing everyday activities

These symptoms could indicate a more serious condition that requires professional evaluation.

Lower back stretches are a powerful tool in managing pain, enhancing flexibility, and improving overall mobility. By integrating these stretches into your daily routine, you can foster a greater sense of well-being and enjoy a more active, fulfilling life. Remember that consistency is key; the more regularly you practice these stretches, the more benefits you will reap. Embrace the journey toward a healthier, more flexible you, and enjoy the newfound freedom of movement that comes with it.

Hip Flexor Stretch

Understanding the Hip Flexors
The hip flexors are a group of muscles located at the front of your hips. They play a crucial role in everyday movements, including walking, running, sitting, and standing. The primary muscles in this group include the iliopsoas, rectus femoris, and sartorius. When these muscles become tight or overactive—often due to prolonged sitting or repetitive activities—they can lead to discomfort, reduced mobility, and even lower back pain.

Regularly stretching your hip flexors can help alleviate these issues, improve your range of motion, and enhance your overall physical performance.

Benefits of Stretching the Hip Flexors
Before diving into the stretch itself, let's explore some of the numerous benefits:

Improved Flexibility: Regular stretching of the hip flexors increases their length, enhancing your overall flexibility and making it easier to perform a variety of movements.

Enhanced Posture: Tight hip flexors can lead to a forward pelvic tilt, resulting in poor posture. Stretching these muscles helps realign your pelvis and spine, promoting better posture.

Reduced Risk of Injury: Flexible hip flexors can reduce the strain on your lower back and pelvis during physical activities, lowering your risk of injury, especially in sports that involve running or jumping.

Better Athletic Performance: Increased hip mobility contributes to more powerful and efficient movements, benefiting activities such as running, cycling, and dancing.

Pain Relief: Stretching the hip flexors can relieve tension in the hips and lower back, providing relief from discomfort associated with tightness.

Preparing for the Stretch
Before we begin the hip flexor stretch, it's important to prepare your body:

Warm-Up: Engage in a light warm-up to increase blood flow to your muscles. This can be a brisk walk, gentle marching in place, or dynamic stretches such as leg swings or arm circles for about 5-10 minutes.

Find a Comfortable Space: Choose a flat, soft surface to perform the stretch, such as a yoga mat, carpet, or grass.

Listen to Your Body: Always assess your body's readiness for stretching. If you feel any sharp pain or discomfort, stop and consult a healthcare professional if needed.

The Hip Flexor Stretch: Step-by-Step Guide
1. Start Position: Kneeling Lunge

Kneel on your right knee, ensuring that your left foot is planted firmly in front of you, creating a 90-degree angle with your left knee.
Align your hips so that both hip bones are facing forward, maintaining a straight line from your knee to your ankle.
Engage your core slightly to protect your lower back.
2. Engage Your Glutes

Tuck your pelvis under slightly by engaging your glutes. This small adjustment helps to prevent overarching your lower back during the stretch.
Hold this position for a moment, feeling the stretch begin to activate in the front of your hip on the right side.
3. Stretch the Hip Flexor

Gently push your hips forward. You should begin to feel a stretch in the hip flexor of the right leg. Make sure to keep your torso upright and avoid leaning too far forward.
Raise your right arm (the arm on the same side as your knee) overhead, reaching it toward the ceiling to enhance the stretch. This movement opens up your torso and increases the stretch along your hip flexor.
4. Breathe Deeply

Inhale deeply through your nose, allowing your lungs to fill with air, and hold the stretch for about 15-30 seconds.
As you exhale, sink a little deeper into the stretch, but be careful not to force it. Focus on relaxing into the position.
5. Repeat on the Other Side

Slowly return to the starting position by bringing your right knee back to the floor.
Switch sides by kneeling on your left knee, with your right foot in front of you. Repeat the stretch as described above, ensuring you maintain alignment and engage your core.
Modifications and Variations
If you find it difficult to hold the standard position or if you're working with limited mobility, here are some modifications:

Use a Chair: If kneeling is uncomfortable, you can perform a modified version of this stretch while seated. Sit on the edge of a sturdy chair with your feet flat on the floor. Slide your right leg back behind you while keeping your left foot firmly planted. Lean slightly forward to feel the stretch in your right hip flexor.

Elevate the Back Leg: For a deeper stretch, elevate your back knee on a cushion or a yoga block. This can help provide more length to the hip flexor.

Incorporate a Strap: If you cannot reach your foot or maintain balance, use a strap or towel around the back foot for assistance in holding the position.

Incorporating the Hip Flexor Stretch into Your Routine
To reap the full benefits of the hip flexor stretch, incorporate it into your routine:

Frequency: Aim to perform this stretch 3-4 times a week. After your workouts, stretching will help promote recovery and flexibility.

Hold Time: Gradually work up to holding the stretch for 30-60 seconds, ensuring to maintain your breathing throughout.

Listen to Your Body: If you feel tightness or discomfort, modify the stretch as needed or consult with a fitness professional.

The hip flexor stretch is an essential exercise for maintaining mobility, flexibility, and overall well-being, especially as we age. By regularly incorporating this stretch into your fitness routine, you can combat tightness, improve your posture, and enhance your physical performance.

Remember, consistency is key. Embrace the journey of flexibility, and soon you'll notice the benefits extending far beyond the mat, positively impacting your everyday life.

Seated Hamstring Stretch

Stretching is an essential component of any fitness regimen, especially for seniors seeking to improve flexibility, reduce the risk of injury, and enhance overall mobility. One particularly effective stretch that targets the hamstrings while accommodating varying fitness levels is the Seated Hamstring Stretch. In this detailed guide, we'll explore the benefits, proper technique, variations, and tips for incorporating this stretch into your routine.

Understanding the Hamstrings

Before diving into the seated hamstring stretch, it's essential to understand the hamstrings' role in your body. The hamstrings are a group of three muscles located at the back of your thigh. These muscles are crucial for bending the knee, extending the hip, and aiding in activities such as walking, running, and even sitting.

As we age, the flexibility of these muscles can decline, leading to stiffness, reduced mobility, and increased risk of falls or injuries. Incorporating hamstring stretches into your routine can significantly enhance flexibility, improve posture, and relieve tension in the lower back.

Benefits of the Seated Hamstring Stretch
Improves Flexibility: Regularly performing the seated hamstring stretch can increase the flexibility of your hamstrings, making daily activities like walking and bending easier and more comfortable.

Reduces Lower Back Pain: Tight hamstrings can contribute to lower back pain. This stretch helps alleviate tension, promoting a healthier spine and reducing discomfort.

Enhances Circulation: Stretching increases blood flow to the muscles, which can improve circulation and help your body recover from workouts more effectively.

Promotes Relaxation: Taking the time to stretch can also serve as a mindful practice, helping to reduce stress and improve overall mental well-being.

Prevents Injuries: By increasing flexibility and range of motion, the seated hamstring stretch can help prevent strains and injuries during physical activity.

Performing the Seated Hamstring Stretch
1. Preparation:

Find a Comfortable Seat: Choose a sturdy chair or sit on the edge of your bed or a yoga mat. Ensure that the surface is stable to prevent any slips.
Posture: Sit up straight with your feet flat on the floor. Your back should be straight, shoulders relaxed, and head aligned with your spine.
2. Positioning:

Extend one leg straight in front of you, keeping the heel on the ground and the toes pointing upward. Bend the opposite knee so that your foot remains flat on the floor.
If you prefer, you can perform the stretch with both legs extended, but be cautious and only do this if you feel comfortable and stable.
3. Stretching Technique:

Inhale deeply and lengthen your spine. Imagine creating space between each vertebra.

Exhale as you gently lean forward from your hips toward the extended leg. Keep your back straight and avoid rounding your shoulders.

Reach for your toes, ankle, or shin—wherever you can comfortably reach without straining. It's essential to listen to your body and avoid pushing into pain.

Hold the stretch for 15 to 30 seconds. Focus on your breathing; inhale deeply and exhale slowly, allowing your body to relax into the stretch.

4. Return to Starting Position:

Slowly come back to a seated position by using your hands to support you. Ensure that your back remains straight as you rise.

Switch legs and repeat the stretch on the opposite side.

5. Frequency:

Aim to perform the seated hamstring stretch 2 to 3 times a week for optimal results. As you become more flexible, you may increase the duration of the stretch to 30 to 60 seconds.

Modifications and Variations

Everyone's body is different, and some seniors may find it challenging to reach their toes or feel discomfort during the stretch. Here are a few modifications to consider:

Use a Strap or Towel: If you can't reach your foot, loop a strap or towel around the ball of your foot to gently pull your leg closer while keeping your back straight.

Perform the Stretch with a Bend: If you experience tightness in your hamstrings, you can perform the stretch with a slight bend in your knee. This modification can reduce tension while still providing benefits.

Add a Twist: For an added stretch, after leaning forward, gently twist your torso toward the extended leg. This variation targets your lower back and promotes spinal mobility.

Tips for Success

Warm-Up First: Always perform a brief warm-up before stretching. Simple movements like marching in place or gentle arm circles can prepare your muscles for stretching.

Focus on Breathing: Deep breathing helps to relax your muscles and enhances the stretch. Inhale through your nose, allowing your abdomen to expand, and exhale through your mouth.

Avoid Bouncing: Stretching should be a gentle, controlled movement. Avoid bouncing or jerking motions, as this can lead to injury.

Listen to Your Body: If you experience pain or discomfort beyond a mild stretch, ease off. It's essential to distinguish between discomfort and pain.

Incorporate into Routine: Consider adding the seated hamstring stretch to your daily routine, especially after activities that involve sitting for extended periods.

The Seated Hamstring Stretch is a valuable addition to any senior's fitness routine, promoting flexibility, reducing pain, and enhancing overall quality of life. By taking the time to incorporate this simple yet effective stretch, you can help maintain mobility and independence as you age.

Remember, the key to successful stretching is consistency, patience, and mindfulness. As you become more comfortable with the seated hamstring stretch, you'll likely notice improvements not only in your hamstring flexibility but also in your overall physical and mental well-being. Embrace this practice, and enjoy the journey toward a healthier, more active lifestyle!

Building a Stretching Routine for Flexibility and Pain Prevention

For seniors over 60, regular stretching not only enhances flexibility but also plays a crucial role in preventing pain and reducing the risk of injuries. This comprehensive guide will help you build a personalized stretching routine tailored to your needs, allowing you to move with ease and comfort.

Understanding the Importance of Stretching
Stretching is often overlooked in exercise regimens, but its benefits cannot be overstated. Here are several reasons why incorporating a consistent stretching routine is essential for seniors:

Enhanced Flexibility: Flexibility is the range of motion available at a joint. With age, tendons and ligaments can become stiffer, leading to decreased flexibility. Regular stretching helps maintain and even improve this range of motion, making daily activities easier.

Pain Prevention: Tight muscles and connective tissues can contribute to chronic pain, especially in the neck, back, and joints. Stretching can alleviate tension and improve blood circulation, reducing the likelihood of pain and discomfort.

Improved Posture: Many seniors struggle with poor posture, which can lead to back pain and other issues. Stretching the chest, shoulders, and hip flexors can counteract the effects of slouching and promote a healthier posture.

Enhanced Performance in Daily Activities: Flexibility allows for greater ease in performing everyday tasks such as bending down to tie shoes, reaching for items on high shelves, or even walking without stiffness.

Stress Relief: Stretching not only benefits the body but also the mind. Incorporating deep breathing and mindfulness into your stretching routine can reduce stress levels and promote relaxation.

Designing Your Stretching Routine
Building a stretching routine tailored to your needs involves several steps. Follow this guide to create a safe and effective program.

Step 1: Assess Your Flexibility Needs
Before starting any new exercise routine, it's important to assess your current flexibility levels. Pay attention to which areas of your body feel tight or restricted. Common areas of tightness for seniors include:

Neck and shoulders
Back
Hips
Hamstrings
Calves
You might consider performing some gentle stretches to gauge your current flexibility levels, noting any discomfort or limitations.

Step 2: Choose the Right Time and Space
Find a quiet, comfortable space in your home where you can focus on stretching. This might be a living room, a dedicated exercise area, or even outside in a garden. The ideal time to stretch is when your muscles are warm, so consider stretching after light activities like walking or after a short warm-up.

Step 3: Warm-Up
Before you begin stretching, it's essential to warm up your body. A gentle warm-up increases blood flow to the muscles and prepares them for stretching. Here's a simple warm-up routine you can follow:

March in Place: 2-3 minutes of marching can get your blood circulating.

Arm Circles: Stand or sit with your arms extended. Make small circles with your arms, gradually increasing the size. Do this for 30 seconds in each direction.

Neck Rolls: Slowly roll your head in a circular motion, first clockwise and then counterclockwise for about 30 seconds.

Step 4: Start Stretching

Now it's time to dive into the stretching routine. Aim for a balanced approach, targeting all major muscle groups. Here are some stretches specifically designed for seniors, focusing on flexibility and pain prevention:

Neck Stretch

Sit or stand comfortably.
Slowly tilt your head to the right, bringing your ear toward your shoulder.
Hold for 15-30 seconds, feeling the stretch along the left side of your neck.
Repeat on the left side.
Shoulder Stretch

Bring your right arm across your chest.
Use your left hand to gently pull your right arm closer to your body.
Hold for 15-30 seconds, then switch arms.
Chest Opener

Stand or sit with your back straight.
Clasp your hands behind your back and gently lift your arms away from your body.
Hold for 15-30 seconds while breathing deeply, feeling the stretch across your chest.
Upper Back Stretch

Sit in a chair with your feet flat on the floor.
Interlace your fingers and stretch your arms forward, rounding your back.
Hold for 15-30 seconds.
Torso Twist

Sit with your feet flat and shoulder-width apart.
Place your right hand on the back of your chair and gently twist your torso to the right.
Hold for 15-30 seconds, then repeat on the left side.
Hip Flexor Stretch

Stand and take a step back with your right leg, bending your left knee.
Keep your right leg straight and press your hips forward.

Hold for 15-30 seconds, then switch legs.
Hamstring Stretch

Sit on the edge of a chair, straightening one leg in front of you.
Keep your knee slightly bent and reach toward your toes.
Hold for 15-30 seconds, feeling the stretch in the back of your thigh.
Calf Stretch

Stand facing a wall, placing your hands against it.
Step back with one foot, keeping it straight and bending your front knee.
Hold for 15-30 seconds, then switch legs.
Ankle Rolls

While seated, lift one foot off the ground and rotate your ankle clockwise, then counterclockwise.
Perform for 30 seconds on each foot.
Step 5: Cool Down
After completing your stretching routine, take a moment to cool down. Stand or sit quietly, focusing on your breath. Inhale deeply through your nose and exhale slowly through your mouth. This practice helps relax your body and mind.

Step 6: Frequency and Progression
Aim to perform your stretching routine at least 2-3 times a week, though daily practice is ideal. As you become more comfortable, gradually increase the duration of each stretch, holding them for longer periods or incorporating new stretches into your routine.

Listening to Your Body
Always listen to your body while stretching. You should feel a gentle pull in the muscle, but never pain. If a stretch causes discomfort, ease out of it and adjust your position. It's crucial to respect your body's limits and progress at your own pace.

Additional Tips for Success
Stay Hydrated: Drink plenty of water before and after your stretching routine to keep your muscles hydrated.
Incorporate Breathing: Focus on your breath throughout your routine. Deep, controlled breathing can enhance the effectiveness of your stretches and promote relaxation.
Consider a Partner: If possible, involve a family member or friend in your stretching routine. This not only makes it more enjoyable but can also provide motivation and support.
Use Props: Don't hesitate to use a towel, strap, or even a belt to assist with stretches. These can help you achieve deeper stretches safely.

Set Realistic Goals: Progress may be slow, and that's perfectly normal. Celebrate small victories and aim for consistency rather than perfection.

Building a stretching routine is a powerful step toward enhancing flexibility and preventing pain, especially as we age. By dedicating time to stretching, you're investing in your long-term health, ensuring that you remain active and engaged in life's activities. Remember that flexibility takes time to develop, so be patient with yourself as you work toward your goals. Embrace the journey, and enjoy the benefits of a more flexible, pain-free life.

Chapter 6: A Balanced Diet to Support Weight Loss and Fitness Goals

Nutrition Basics for Seniors: Supporting an Active Lifestyle

For seniors, particularly those over 60, a well-balanced diet is crucial not just for maintaining weight, but also for enhancing overall health, preventing chronic diseases, and supporting an active lifestyle. In this chapter, we will delve into the fundamental aspects of nutrition for seniors, addressing what they need to thrive.

Understanding the Role of Nutrition
Nutrition is more than just fuel for the body; it's the foundation of health. Proper nutrition helps seniors maintain muscle mass, bone density, and cognitive function. It can also mitigate the risk of chronic conditions such as heart disease, diabetes, and osteoporosis. The right balance of nutrients can significantly enhance quality of life, ensuring that seniors can engage in daily activities, exercise, and enjoy their hobbies without physical limitations.

Key Nutritional Components
Macronutrients: Carbohydrates, Proteins, and Fats

Carbohydrates: Often vilified in trendy diets, carbohydrates are essential for energy, particularly for seniors who lead active lives. Choose complex carbohydrates, such as whole grains, legumes, fruits, and vegetables. These options provide sustained energy and are rich in fiber, which aids digestion and helps maintain stable blood sugar levels.

Proteins: As muscle mass naturally declines with age, adequate protein intake becomes vital for preserving muscle strength and function. Seniors should aim for lean protein sources such as chicken, turkey, fish, eggs, dairy products, legumes, and plant-based proteins like quinoa and tofu. Aiming for 1.0 to 1.2 grams of protein per kilogram of body weight daily is a good target for older adults.

Fats: Healthy fats are essential for heart health and cognitive function. Incorporate sources of unsaturated fats, such as avocados, nuts, seeds, olive oil, and fatty fish like salmon. These fats can help lower cholesterol levels and support overall cardiovascular health.

Micronutrients: Vitamins and Minerals

Calcium and Vitamin D: Bone health is a significant concern for seniors. Calcium is crucial for maintaining bone density, while vitamin D helps the body absorb calcium. Dairy products, leafy greens, fortified foods, and fatty fish are excellent sources. Regular sun exposure can also help boost vitamin D levels, but supplements may be necessary for those with limited sun exposure.

B Vitamins: B vitamins, including B12 and folate, play critical roles in energy metabolism and brain health. Seniors often have reduced absorption of vitamin B12 due to changes in stomach acid production. Sources include meat, eggs, dairy products, and fortified cereals. Dark leafy greens and legumes provide folate, which is important for cell division and overall health.

Antioxidants: Vitamins C and E, along with minerals like selenium, act as antioxidants, helping to combat oxidative stress and inflammation. Fresh fruits and vegetables, nuts, seeds, and whole grains are rich in these essential nutrients. Aim for a rainbow of produce to ensure a wide range of antioxidants in your diet.

Hydration

Staying hydrated is essential for all ages, but it becomes increasingly important as we age. Seniors often have a diminished sense of thirst and may not drink enough fluids, leading to dehydration. Adequate hydration supports digestion, helps regulate body temperature, and aids in cognitive function. Aim for at least 8 cups of fluids a day, and remember that water isn't the only source. Herbal teas, broths, and hydrating fruits and vegetables (like cucumbers and watermelon) contribute to overall fluid intake.

Special Considerations for Seniors
As we age, various factors can influence our nutritional needs and choices. Here are some key considerations:

Chronic Health Conditions: Seniors may deal with diabetes, hypertension, or heart disease, all of which require careful dietary management. For instance, a low-sodium diet is essential for those with high blood pressure, while diabetics must focus on carbohydrate counting and balanced meals to manage blood sugar levels.

Digestive Health: Aging often comes with changes in digestive health, including a slower metabolism and a higher likelihood of gastrointestinal issues. High-fiber foods such as fruits, vegetables, whole grains, and legumes can help prevent constipation and promote gut health. Probiotic-rich foods, like yogurt and fermented vegetables, can also support digestion.

Taste and Appetite Changes: Seniors may experience changes in taste and smell, leading to decreased appetite. Enhancing the flavor of healthy foods with herbs and spices can make meals more appealing. Eating smaller, more frequent meals rather than three large ones can also help meet nutritional needs without overwhelming the appetite.

Social Factors: Meals are often a social activity, and isolation can lead to poor nutrition. Encouraging communal meals with family or friends, or participating in community dining programs can help combat loneliness and promote healthier eating habits.

Meal Planning for an Active Lifestyle
To support an active lifestyle, seniors should focus on meal planning that is not only nutritious but also enjoyable. Here's how to get started:

Create Balanced Meals: A balanced plate typically consists of half vegetables, a quarter protein, and a quarter whole grains. This formula ensures that meals are nutritionally dense and varied.

Incorporate Snacks: Healthy snacks can help maintain energy levels throughout the day. Opt for nutrient-dense options like nuts, yogurt, fruit, or whole-grain crackers with hummus.

Stay Flexible: While planning is essential, it's also important to stay flexible. Listen to your body's hunger cues and adjust portion sizes and meal timing as needed.

Utilize Meal Prep: Preparing meals in advance can save time and ensure that healthy options are readily available. Consider batch-cooking soups, stews, or casseroles, and portioning them for easy access during the week.

Sample Meal Ideas
To illustrate how to incorporate these nutritional principles into daily life, here are a few sample meal ideas:

Breakfast: Overnight oats made with rolled oats, chia seeds, almond milk, and topped with fresh berries and a sprinkle of nuts.

Lunch: A mixed salad with spinach, cherry tomatoes, cucumber, chickpeas, and grilled chicken, drizzled with olive oil and lemon juice.

Snack: Sliced apple with almond butter or a small handful of mixed nuts.

Dinner: Baked salmon with quinoa and steamed broccoli, seasoned with garlic and herbs.

Dessert: Greek yogurt topped with honey and sliced peaches.

Embracing a well-rounded nutritional approach is fundamental for seniors seeking to lead active, fulfilling lives. By focusing on balanced meals rich in macronutrients and micronutrients, staying hydrated, and considering individual health needs, seniors can optimize their diet to support not only physical health but also mental and emotional well-being.

As you embark on this journey of healthy eating, remember that each small change can lead to significant improvements in your overall quality of life. Stay informed, stay engaged, and most importantly, enjoy the process of nourishing your body!

How Diet Impacts Weight Loss and Energy Levels

Diet plays a critical role in weight loss and overall energy levels, particularly for seniors over 60, who may face unique nutritional challenges and metabolic changes. As a fitness instructor and exercise expert, I often emphasize the connection between what we eat and how we feel. Understanding this relationship can empower individuals to make informed dietary choices that complement their exercise routines and enhance their well-being. Let's delve deeper into how diet impacts weight loss and energy levels, particularly for seniors.

The Connection Between Diet and Weight Loss
Understanding Caloric Balance
At its core, weight loss is about caloric balance. This means that to lose weight, you need to burn more calories than you consume. However, it's not just about eating less; it's also about the quality of those calories. A well-balanced diet should provide essential nutrients while keeping caloric intake in check.

Macronutrients and Their Role
Carbohydrates: Often viewed with suspicion in weight loss discussions, carbohydrates are the body's primary energy source. However, the type of carbs consumed is crucial. Whole grains, fruits, and vegetables are rich in fiber, which helps regulate blood sugar levels and keeps you feeling full longer. In contrast, refined carbs—like white bread and sugary snacks—can lead to spikes in blood sugar followed by crashes, leaving you feeling fatigued and craving more food.

Proteins: Protein is essential for muscle repair and growth, especially important for seniors who want to maintain muscle mass. Including adequate protein in your diet can promote feelings of fullness and reduce overall calorie intake. High-protein foods such as lean meats, fish, eggs, beans, and legumes can help seniors maintain strength and support their exercise goals.

Fats: Healthy fats, such as those found in avocados, nuts, seeds, and olive oil, can also play a role in weight management. Fats are calorie-dense, so moderation is key. However, incorporating healthy fats can help you feel satiated and satisfied, reducing the temptation to snack on less nutritious options.

Portion Control and Mindful Eating

Understanding portion sizes and practicing mindful eating are essential components of a successful weight loss strategy. For seniors, who may have slower metabolisms, it's vital to focus on smaller portions of nutrient-dense foods rather than larger servings of lower-quality options. Mindful eating encourages individuals to pay attention to hunger and fullness cues, which can help prevent overeating.

The Role of Diet in Energy Levels

Nutrient Density and Sustained Energy

The foods we eat directly influence our energy levels. A diet rich in nutrient-dense foods provides the vitamins, minerals, and antioxidants necessary for optimal bodily function. This is especially important for seniors, who may be at risk for deficiencies that can lead to fatigue and decreased energy levels.

Vitamins and Minerals: Micronutrients such as vitamin B12, iron, and magnesium play critical roles in energy production. B12, for example, is essential for red blood cell formation and neurological function. Seniors often struggle to absorb B12, making fortified foods or supplements beneficial. Similarly, iron is crucial for oxygen transport in the blood, and deficiencies can lead to anemia, causing fatigue.

Hydration: Dehydration is a common issue among seniors, leading to decreased energy levels and cognitive function. Water is essential for nearly every bodily function, including digestion and nutrient absorption. Aim to drink at least 8 cups of fluids daily, adjusting for physical activity and individual needs.

Blood Sugar Stability

Consuming a balanced diet helps maintain stable blood sugar levels, which is vital for sustained energy. High-sugar foods can lead to quick spikes in energy followed by sharp crashes, causing fatigue. Instead, focus on a balanced approach that includes fiber-rich foods that slow the absorption of sugar into the bloodstream.

Complex Carbohydrates: Foods like whole grains, legumes, and starchy vegetables provide a gradual release of energy, keeping blood sugar levels stable and energy consistent.

Pairing Foods: Combining carbohydrates with protein and healthy fats can further stabilize blood sugar levels. For instance, pairing apple slices with nut butter provides a satisfying snack that offers both fiber and protein.

Tailoring Your Diet for Weight Loss and Energy
Practical Strategies for Seniors
Focus on Whole Foods: Prioritize whole, unprocessed foods that provide maximum nutrition. These include fruits, vegetables, whole grains, lean proteins, and healthy fats.

Plan and Prepare Meals: Planning meals ahead of time can help avoid last-minute unhealthy choices. Consider batch cooking nutritious meals that can be reheated throughout the week.

Incorporate Variety: Eating a wide range of foods ensures you receive a balanced array of nutrients. Experiment with different fruits, vegetables, and protein sources to keep meals interesting and nutritious.

Listen to Your Body: Pay attention to how different foods make you feel. Keeping a food diary can help identify foods that boost your energy or contribute to feelings of sluggishness.

Small, Frequent Meals: Some seniors find that eating smaller, more frequent meals helps maintain energy levels throughout the day. This approach can prevent the highs and lows associated with larger meals.

Sample Daily Menu
Here's an example of a nutrient-dense daily menu for seniors focused on weight loss and energy:

Breakfast: Oatmeal topped with fresh berries and a sprinkle of nuts, served with a cup of green tea.
Mid-Morning Snack: A small apple with almond butter.
Lunch: Grilled chicken salad with mixed greens, cherry tomatoes, cucumber, and a vinaigrette dressing.
Afternoon Snack: Greek yogurt with a drizzle of honey and a few slices of kiwi.
Dinner: Baked salmon, quinoa, and steamed broccoli.
Evening Snack: A handful of mixed nuts or a small piece of dark chocolate.

In conclusion, diet significantly impacts weight loss and energy levels, particularly for seniors over 60. By focusing on nutrient-dense foods, maintaining proper hydration, and practicing mindful eating, seniors can optimize their health, energy levels, and overall well-being. Remember, making small, sustainable changes to your diet can lead to substantial benefits over time. Pairing these dietary choices with regular chair yoga and strength training exercises can create a holistic approach to health, helping you thrive as you age.

Creating Simple, Healthy Meals

In the journey toward improved health and wellness, nutrition plays an essential role, especially for seniors over 60. As our bodies age, our nutritional needs change, requiring us to be more mindful about the foods we consume. Creating simple, healthy meals doesn't have to be overwhelming. With a few foundational principles, you can prepare delicious dishes that support weight loss, provide energy, and promote overall health.

Understanding Nutritional Needs
Before diving into meal ideas, it's crucial to understand what your body requires. As we age, our metabolism slows down, and our bodies become less efficient at processing certain nutrients. Here are some key points to consider:

Macronutrients:

Proteins: Essential for muscle maintenance and repair. Aim for lean sources like chicken, fish, beans, and legumes.
Carbohydrates: Focus on whole grains, fruits, and vegetables for energy and fiber, which aids digestion.
Fats: Incorporate healthy fats, such as avocados, nuts, seeds, and olive oil, which are vital for brain health and hormone production.
Micronutrients:

Pay attention to vitamins and minerals such as calcium (for bone health), vitamin D (for calcium absorption), and antioxidants found in colorful fruits and vegetables.
Hydration:

Water is often overlooked but is essential for every bodily function. Aim for at least 8 cups of water a day, adjusting based on activity level and climate.
Meal Planning Basics
Planning meals in advance can save time and ensure you have healthy options at hand. Here are some strategies to simplify the process:

Create a Weekly Menu:

Dedicate time each week to plan your meals. Include a variety of proteins, grains, and vegetables to keep meals interesting.

Batch Cooking:

Prepare larger portions of staple ingredients, like grains or proteins, that can be easily mixed and matched throughout the week. For example, cook a big batch of quinoa or brown rice to use in various meals.

Keep It Simple:

Aim for meals that require minimal preparation. Think about one-pot dishes, sheet pan meals, or slow-cooker recipes that allow flavors to meld without much fuss.

Healthy Meal Ideas

Here are several simple meal ideas that combine nutrition, taste, and ease of preparation:

Breakfast Options

Overnight Oats:

Combine rolled oats with yogurt or milk, chia seeds, and your favorite fruits. Leave it in the fridge overnight, and grab it in the morning for a quick, nutritious breakfast.

Veggie Omelette:

Whisk eggs with a splash of milk, pour into a heated non-stick pan, and add diced vegetables such as spinach, bell peppers, and onions. Cook until set and serve with whole-grain toast.

Smoothie Bowl:

Blend a banana, a handful of spinach, and a cup of frozen berries with almond milk. Pour it into a bowl and top with sliced fruits, nuts, and seeds for added crunch.

Lunch Ideas

Quinoa Salad:

Toss cooked quinoa with chopped cucumbers, cherry tomatoes, bell peppers, and a simple vinaigrette made of olive oil, lemon juice, salt, and pepper. Add chickpeas or grilled chicken for extra protein.

Lentil Soup:

Simmer lentils with diced carrots, celery, onions, and garlic in vegetable broth. Season with herbs like thyme and bay leaves. This hearty soup is packed with protein and fiber.

Wraps:

Use whole-grain tortillas to wrap sliced turkey, spinach, avocado, and hummus. This is an easy, portable meal that's high in protein and healthy fats.

Dinner Dishes

Sheet Pan Salmon and Vegetables:

Place salmon fillets on a sheet pan with broccoli and sweet potatoes. Drizzle with olive oil, lemon juice, and your favorite seasonings. Roast in the oven until the salmon flakes easily.

Stir-Fried Vegetables and Tofu:

Sauté a mix of colorful vegetables (bell peppers, carrots, snap peas) with cubed tofu in a bit of sesame oil and soy sauce. Serve over brown rice or quinoa.

Stuffed Bell Peppers:

Fill halved bell peppers with a mixture of cooked ground turkey, black beans, corn, and brown rice. Top with a sprinkle of cheese and bake until the peppers are tender.

Snack Suggestions

Greek Yogurt with Honey and Nuts:

A protein-rich snack that satisfies sweet cravings. Top Greek yogurt with a drizzle of honey and a handful of mixed nuts or seeds.

Veggie Sticks with Hummus:

Cut up carrots, cucumbers, and bell peppers to dip into hummus. This combination provides fiber and healthy fats.

Air-Popped Popcorn:

A low-calorie snack when seasoned with spices instead of butter. Sprinkle with nutritional yeast for a cheesy flavor.

Tips for Healthy Cooking

Use Fresh Ingredients: Whenever possible, use fresh vegetables and fruits. They offer more nutrients and flavor compared to processed options.

Mindful Cooking: Take your time when preparing meals. Enjoy the process of chopping, stirring, and tasting. This mindfulness can improve your relationship with food.

Experiment with Herbs and Spices: These can enhance flavor without adding extra calories or sodium. Try basil, oregano, rosemary, turmeric, and ginger to give your meals a boost.

Limit Processed Foods: They often contain high levels of sodium, sugars, and unhealthy fats. Focus on whole, minimally processed ingredients.

Building a Healthy Plate
To create balanced meals, aim to fill half your plate with fruits and vegetables, a quarter with whole grains, and a quarter with protein. This method helps ensure that you're getting a variety of nutrients while keeping portion sizes in check.

Creating simple, healthy meals is a cornerstone of maintaining health and vitality after 60. By understanding your nutritional needs and embracing easy, nutritious recipes, you can transform your diet and support your exercise goals. Remember, the journey to better health is gradual, so celebrate each small victory and stay committed to your wellness. With these tips and meal ideas, you'll be well on your way to enjoying delicious, healthful eating that complements your active lifestyle.

Recipes for Weight Loss and Energy

Low-Carb Meals

In the pursuit of weight loss and enhanced energy levels, dietary choices play a pivotal role, particularly as we age. For seniors over 60, embracing low-carb meals can lead to significant benefits, including weight management, improved blood sugar levels, and sustained energy throughout the day. This chapter will guide you through a variety of low-carb recipes that are not only nutritious and satisfying but also easy to prepare. These meals are designed to be delicious and supportive of your fitness goals, allowing you to enjoy flavorful dishes while keeping your carbohydrate intake in check.

Understanding Low-Carb Eating
Before diving into the recipes, let's explore the fundamentals of a low-carb diet. The essence of low-carb eating is to reduce the intake of foods that are high in sugars and starches, replacing them with nutrient-dense options. This shift can help your body enter a state of ketosis, where it begins to burn fat for fuel instead of carbohydrates. The benefits of low-carb meals for seniors can include:

Weight Loss: Lowering carbohydrate intake can reduce insulin levels, leading to increased fat burning.
Enhanced Energy: By stabilizing blood sugar levels, low-carb diets can provide sustained energy without the crashes associated with high-carb meals.
Improved Heart Health: Reducing carb intake can help lower cholesterol levels and improve overall heart health, which is crucial as we age.

With this understanding, let's delve into some easy and flavorful low-carb recipes that you can incorporate into your weekly meal plan.

Recipe 1: Zucchini Noodles with Pesto and Grilled Chicken
Ingredients:
2 medium zucchinis, spiralized
1 cup cherry tomatoes, halved
1 cup basil pesto (store-bought or homemade)
2 boneless, skinless chicken breasts
2 tablespoons olive oil
Salt and pepper, to taste
Grated Parmesan cheese, for serving (optional)
Instructions:
Prepare the Chicken: Preheat your grill or stovetop grill pan over medium-high heat. Season the chicken breasts with olive oil, salt, and pepper. Grill the chicken for 6-7 minutes on each side, or until cooked through. Remove from heat and let it rest for a few minutes before slicing.

Make the Zucchini Noodles: In a large skillet, heat a tablespoon of olive oil over medium heat. Add the spiralized zucchini and sauté for about 2-3 minutes, just until slightly tender but still firm. Season with salt and pepper.

Combine: In a bowl, toss the sautéed zucchini noodles with pesto and halved cherry tomatoes. Add the sliced grilled chicken on top.

Serve: Garnish with grated Parmesan cheese if desired. This dish is not only low in carbs but also packed with flavor and healthy fats from the pesto.

Recipe 2: Cauliflower Fried Rice
Ingredients:
- 1 medium head of cauliflower, riced (or 4 cups pre-riced cauliflower)
- 1 cup mixed vegetables (peas, carrots, bell peppers)
- 2 large eggs, beaten
- 3 green onions, sliced
- 2 tablespoons soy sauce or tamari
- 1 tablespoon sesame oil
- 2 cloves garlic, minced
- Salt and pepper, to taste

Instructions:
Prepare the Cauliflower Rice: If using a whole head of cauliflower, remove the leaves and stem. Cut it into florets and pulse in a food processor until it resembles rice.

Cook the Eggs: In a large skillet or wok, heat sesame oil over medium heat. Add the beaten eggs and scramble until fully cooked. Remove the eggs from the skillet and set aside.

Stir-Fry Vegetables: In the same skillet, add garlic and mixed vegetables. Sauté for 3-4 minutes until vegetables are tender.

Add Cauliflower Rice: Stir in the riced cauliflower and soy sauce. Cook for another 5-7 minutes, stirring frequently, until the cauliflower is tender but not mushy.

Combine: Return the scrambled eggs to the skillet, add green onions, and mix well. Season with salt and pepper to taste.

Serve: This cauliflower fried rice is a fantastic low-carb alternative to traditional fried rice, providing a satisfying and nutritious meal.

Recipe 3: Egg and Spinach Breakfast Muffins
Ingredients:
- 6 large eggs
- 1 cup fresh spinach, chopped
- 1/2 cup diced bell peppers (any color)
- 1/4 cup feta cheese, crumbled (optional)
- Salt and pepper, to taste
- Cooking spray or oil for greasing the muffin tin

Instructions:
Preheat the Oven: Preheat your oven to 350°F (175°C) and grease a muffin tin with cooking spray or oil.

Mix Ingredients: In a large bowl, whisk the eggs until well combined. Stir in chopped spinach, bell peppers, feta cheese (if using), and season with salt and pepper.

Fill Muffin Tin: Pour the egg mixture evenly into the muffin tin, filling each cup about 2/3 full.

Bake: Bake for 18-20 minutes or until the eggs are set and slightly golden on top.

Cool and Serve: Let the muffins cool for a few minutes before removing them from the tin. These muffins can be stored in the refrigerator for up to a week and are perfect for a quick breakfast on the go.

Recipe 4: Grilled Salmon with Asparagus

Ingredients:
2 salmon fillets
1 bunch asparagus, trimmed
2 tablespoons olive oil
Juice of 1 lemon
2 cloves garlic, minced
Salt and pepper, to taste
Fresh dill or parsley for garnish (optional)

Instructions:

Prepare the Marinade: In a small bowl, whisk together olive oil, lemon juice, minced garlic, salt, and pepper.

Marinate Salmon: Place the salmon fillets in a shallow dish and pour half of the marinade over them. Let marinate for at least 15 minutes.

Grill the Salmon and Asparagus: Preheat your grill or grill pan over medium-high heat. Grill the salmon skin-side down for about 5-6 minutes. Add the asparagus to the grill and cook for 3-4 minutes, turning occasionally until tender and slightly charred.

Serve: Plate the grilled salmon and asparagus, drizzling the remaining marinade over the top. Garnish with fresh dill or parsley if desired. This meal is rich in omega-3 fatty acids and packed with nutrients, making it ideal for weight loss and energy.

Tips for Success with Low-Carb Meals

Plan Your Meals: Take time each week to plan your low-carb meals. This helps ensure you have all the ingredients on hand and reduces the temptation to reach for high-carb options.

Experiment with Spices: Low-carb meals don't have to be bland. Use various herbs and spices to enhance flavor without adding carbs.

Stay Hydrated: Drinking plenty of water is essential when following a low-carb diet. It aids digestion and can help control hunger.

Listen to Your Body: Pay attention to how different foods affect your energy levels and overall well-being. Adjust your meals accordingly.

Low-carb meals can be delicious, satisfying, and highly beneficial for weight loss and energy, especially for seniors over 60. By incorporating these recipes into your diet, you'll not only enjoy a variety of flavors but also support your fitness journey. Remember, the goal is not only to lose weight but also to gain energy and enhance your overall quality of life. So, get cooking, savor these meals, and embrace the wonderful benefits of a low-carb lifestyle!

High-Protein Snacks

As we age, especially for seniors over 60, our nutritional needs evolve, and maintaining a balanced diet becomes increasingly crucial. One important aspect of this diet is protein, which plays a vital role in muscle repair, immune function, and overall health. High-protein snacks can be an excellent way to ensure you meet your daily protein requirements without feeling overly full or bogged down by heavy meals. In this guide, we'll explore the benefits of high-protein snacks, provide a variety of options, and offer tips for incorporating them into your daily routine.

Understanding the Importance of Protein
Protein is one of the three macronutrients essential for our bodies, alongside carbohydrates and fats. It is made up of amino acids, which are the building blocks of our cells. As we age, our bodies become less efficient at synthesizing protein, making it essential to consume adequate amounts through our diet. Here are some of the key benefits of maintaining a high-protein diet, particularly for seniors:

1. Muscle Maintenance and Repair
After 60, muscle mass naturally begins to decline, a condition known as sarcopenia. Consuming high-protein snacks helps counteract this muscle loss by providing the necessary building blocks for muscle repair and growth. This is particularly important for maintaining strength, balance, and mobility.

2. Satiety and Weight Management
Protein is known to increase feelings of fullness and satisfaction. Including high-protein snacks in your diet can help curb hunger pangs, making it easier to manage your weight. This is especially beneficial for those looking to lose or maintain weight as they age.

3. Bone Health
Many protein sources, particularly animal-based ones, are rich in calcium and other nutrients that support bone health. Adequate protein intake has been associated with improved bone density, reducing the risk of fractures and osteoporosis.

4. Enhanced Recovery
For seniors engaging in physical activity, protein is crucial for recovery. It aids in repairing muscle tissue after exercise, reducing soreness, and preparing the body for future workouts.

5. Improved Immune Function
Protein plays a critical role in the immune system, helping to produce antibodies and other immune factors. A diet rich in protein can help keep your immune system strong, especially important for seniors who may be more susceptible to infections.

Choosing the Right High-Protein Snacks

When selecting snacks, it's important to choose options that are not only high in protein but also low in added sugars, unhealthy fats, and excessive sodium. Here are some excellent choices for high-protein snacks that are both nutritious and easy to prepare:

1. Greek Yogurt

Greek yogurt is a fantastic source of protein, offering about 15-20 grams per serving. It's also rich in probiotics, which support gut health. For added flavor and nutrition, top it with fresh berries, nuts, or a drizzle of honey.

2. Cottage Cheese

Cottage cheese is another high-protein dairy option, packing around 14 grams of protein in just half a cup. It's versatile and can be enjoyed on its own or mixed with fruits, vegetables, or whole-grain crackers for a balanced snack.

3. Hard-Boiled Eggs

Eggs are a powerhouse of nutrition, providing about 6 grams of protein each. Hard-boiled eggs are easy to prepare in advance and make for a portable snack. Sprinkle them with a little salt, pepper, or your favorite seasoning for a quick protein boost.

4. Nuts and Seeds

While nuts and seeds are higher in calories, they are also rich in protein and healthy fats. Almonds, walnuts, pumpkin seeds, and chia seeds offer about 5-7 grams of protein per ounce. A small handful makes a satisfying snack. Just be mindful of portion sizes.

5. Edamame

These young soybeans are not only a good source of protein (about 17 grams per cup) but also high in fiber and various vitamins. Steam them lightly and sprinkle with sea salt for a delicious and nutritious snack.

6. Protein Bars

When choosing protein bars, look for those with minimal added sugars and natural ingredients. They typically offer 10-20 grams of protein per bar and can be a convenient option for on-the-go snacking.

7. Jerky

Beef, turkey, or chicken jerky can be a great high-protein snack, with about 9 grams of protein per ounce. Opt for lower-sodium versions and be cautious about added preservatives.

8. Hummus with Veggies

Hummus, made from chickpeas, offers about 5 grams of protein per serving. Pair it with carrot sticks, cucumber slices, or bell pepper strips for a crunchy, nutritious snack that's high in fiber as well.

9. Protein Smoothies

Smoothies are a great way to pack in protein and nutrients. Blend a scoop of protein powder (whey, pea, or soy) with your favorite fruits, vegetables, and a base of yogurt or milk for a delicious and filling snack.

10. Chickpea Salad

Chickpeas are a fantastic plant-based protein source, providing about 7 grams of protein per half-cup. Toss them with diced vegetables, olive oil, lemon juice, and herbs for a refreshing and protein-rich salad.

Incorporating High-Protein Snacks into Your Day

To reap the benefits of high-protein snacks, consider these strategies for incorporating them into your daily routine:

1. Plan Ahead

Preparation is key. Set aside time each week to prepare snacks in advance, such as hard-boiling eggs, portioning nuts, or making a batch of protein bars. This makes it easier to grab healthy options when hunger strikes.

2. Pair Protein with Other Nutrients

For optimal nutrition, pair your high-protein snacks with carbohydrates and healthy fats. For example, enjoy Greek yogurt with fruit and nuts or hummus with veggies. This balance can help keep your energy levels steady.

3. Listen to Your Body

Pay attention to your hunger cues. Incorporate high-protein snacks between meals to stave off hunger and avoid overeating during meal times. Aim for snacks that keep you satisfied until your next meal.

4. Experiment with Recipes

Try different combinations and recipes to keep things interesting. Explore protein-rich smoothie recipes or create your own nut butter blends. Get creative with flavors and textures to make healthy snacking enjoyable.

5. Stay Hydrated

Don't forget to drink plenty of water throughout the day. Hydration is essential for overall health, and it can also help prevent confusion between hunger and thirst.

High-protein snacks can be a vital component of a balanced diet for seniors over 60, supporting muscle health, weight management, and overall well-being. By selecting nutrient-dense options and incorporating them into your daily routine, you can enjoy the many benefits protein has to offer. Whether it's a serving of Greek yogurt, a handful of nuts, or a delicious chickpea salad, these snacks not only provide essential nutrients but also keep you energized and satisfied throughout the day. Embrace these delicious and healthy choices as part of your journey to maintaining a vibrant, active lifestyle as you age.

Anti-Inflammatory Smoothies

In recent years, the emphasis on nutrition has expanded beyond mere calorie counting and macronutrient balancing. Now more than ever, individuals are becoming aware of how certain foods can either promote health or contribute to inflammation—a key factor in numerous chronic diseases. Anti-inflammatory smoothies offer a refreshing and nutritious way to combat inflammation while providing a wealth of vitamins, minerals, and antioxidants.

Understanding Inflammation
Before diving into the world of smoothies, it's essential to understand what inflammation is and why it matters. Inflammation is a natural response by the body's immune system to injury or infection. Acute inflammation, which occurs after an injury or infection, is beneficial. However, chronic inflammation—persistent inflammation that can last for months or years—has been linked to various health conditions, including arthritis, heart disease, diabetes, and certain cancers.

Foods rich in antioxidants, omega-3 fatty acids, and specific vitamins can help reduce inflammation in the body. Anti-inflammatory smoothies are a fantastic way to incorporate these foods into your diet, allowing for easy digestion and absorption of nutrients.

The Benefits of Anti-Inflammatory Smoothies
Nutrient-Dense: Smoothies can be packed with nutrient-dense ingredients, providing a variety of vitamins and minerals in one meal or snack.

Easy to Digest: Blending breaks down the cell walls of fruits and vegetables, making it easier for your body to absorb nutrients. This is especially beneficial for seniors or those with digestive issues.

Hydrating: Smoothies often contain water-rich fruits and vegetables, helping to keep you hydrated.

Customizable: You can tailor your smoothie to your taste preferences and nutritional needs, experimenting with different flavors and ingredients.

Quick and Convenient: Preparing a smoothie takes just a few minutes, making it an ideal option for busy individuals or those who need a quick meal on the go.

Key Ingredients for Anti-Inflammatory Smoothies
When crafting your anti-inflammatory smoothies, focus on incorporating the following key ingredients:

Fruits:

Berries (blueberries, strawberries, raspberries, blackberries): These are high in antioxidants and vitamins, particularly vitamin C, which can help reduce inflammation.
Pineapple: Contains bromelain, an enzyme known for its anti-inflammatory properties.
Bananas: Provide potassium and other nutrients, helping to balance electrolytes and support overall health.
Vegetables:

Spinach: Packed with antioxidants, vitamins A and C, and flavonoids that help combat inflammation.
Kale: Another leafy green high in antioxidants and vitamins. Kale can also provide fiber, which is beneficial for gut health.
Beets: Rich in nitrates and antioxidants, beets can help reduce inflammation and improve blood flow.

Healthy Fats:

Avocado: High in monounsaturated fats and vitamins E and C, avocados help lower inflammation while adding creaminess to your smoothie.
Nut Butters (almond, walnut, or peanut butter): These provide healthy fats and proteins, making your smoothie more filling and nutritious.
Seeds:

Chia Seeds: Loaded with omega-3 fatty acids and fiber, chia seeds are excellent for reducing inflammation and promoting digestive health.
Flaxseeds: Another source of omega-3s, flaxseeds are particularly beneficial for heart health.

Liquid Bases:

Coconut Water: A hydrating base that is rich in electrolytes, coconut water adds a tropical flavor while supporting hydration.
Almond Milk or Coconut Milk: These dairy alternatives are often lower in calories and can be enriched with vitamins and minerals.
Spices:

Turmeric: Known for its powerful anti-inflammatory properties, turmeric contains curcumin, which can be enhanced when combined with black pepper for better absorption.
Ginger: This root has been shown to reduce inflammation and improve digestion. Fresh ginger can add a zesty kick to your smoothie.
Sample Anti-Inflammatory Smoothie Recipes
Now that we have a solid understanding of the key ingredients, let's explore some delicious anti-inflammatory smoothie recipes that you can easily prepare at home.

1. Berry Bliss Smoothie
Ingredients:

- 1 cup mixed berries (blueberries, strawberries, raspberries)
- 1 banana
- 1 cup spinach
- 1 tablespoon chia seeds
- 1 cup almond milk (or coconut water)
- 1 teaspoon honey (optional)

Instructions:

Place all ingredients in a blender.
Blend until smooth and creamy. Add more liquid if necessary to reach your desired consistency.
Taste and adjust sweetness with honey if desired.
Benefits: This smoothie is packed with antioxidants from the berries and vitamins from the spinach, along with the healthy fats from chia seeds.

2. Tropical Turmeric Smoothie
Ingredients:

- 1 cup pineapple chunks (fresh or frozen)
- 1 banana
- 1 teaspoon grated fresh ginger

- 1 teaspoon ground turmeric
- 1 cup coconut milk
- Pinch of black pepper (to enhance turmeric absorption)

Instructions:

Combine all ingredients in a blender.
Blend until smooth. You can add ice for a colder, thicker texture.
Serve immediately.
Benefits: This tropical smoothie not only tastes great but also leverages the anti-inflammatory benefits of turmeric and ginger.

3. Green Goddess Smoothie
Ingredients:

- 1 cup kale (stems removed)
- 1 cup cucumber (peeled and chopped)
- 1 avocado
- 1 tablespoon flaxseeds
- 1 tablespoon lemon juice
- 1 cup water or coconut water

Instructions:

Add all ingredients to a blender.
Blend until creamy and smooth, adjusting the liquid to achieve your desired consistency.
Enjoy as a refreshing meal or snack.
Benefits: This smoothie is full of healthy fats from the avocado and provides a host of vitamins from the greens, making it perfect for anti-inflammatory benefits.

Tips for Crafting the Perfect Anti-Inflammatory Smoothie
Balance Flavors: Aim for a good mix of sweet, tart, and creamy flavors. Fruits can add natural sweetness, while leafy greens provide a fresh taste.

Experiment with Textures: Some people prefer thicker smoothies, while others like them thinner. Adjust the liquid content accordingly.

Blend in Steps: If using tougher ingredients like frozen fruits or vegetables, blend them first with a bit of liquid before adding softer ingredients.

Stay Seasonal: Using seasonal fruits and vegetables not only ensures better taste but also supports local farmers and reduces environmental impact.

Prep Ahead: Make smoothie packs by portioning ingredients into freezer bags. Just grab a bag in the morning, add your liquid, and blend!

Incorporating anti-inflammatory smoothies into your diet is not just about reducing inflammation; it's about embracing a lifestyle of wellness, vitality, and flavor. These delicious concoctions serve as a testament to the power of whole foods, reminding us that health can be enjoyable. With a little creativity and the right ingredients, smoothies can become an integral part of your daily routine, helping you feel energized and revitalized.

Remember, while smoothies are a great addition to a healthy diet, they are most effective when combined with a balanced diet, regular physical activity, and adequate hydration. So, blend your way to better health and enjoy every sip!

Chapter 7: Putting It All Together: A 4-Week Exercise Plan

Week 1: Getting Acquainted with Movement

Sample Weekly Schedule:

Days	Activity
Monday	Chair Yoga Session
Tuesday	Upper Body Strength Training
Wednesday	Lower Body Strength Training
Thursday	Chair Yoga Session
Friday	Body Stretch and Light Cardio
Saturday	Rest Day
Sunday	Rest Day

Welcome to Week 1 of your journey toward improved health and well-being! This week is all about gently introducing your body to movement, allowing you to reconnect with your physical capabilities. Whether you're coming back from a long hiatus or just beginning your exercise journey, this week will set a solid foundation for the weeks to come. Let's dive into the structure of this week, focusing on simple movements that promote flexibility, strength, and overall vitality.

Understanding Your Body's Needs
Before we jump into the exercises, it's essential to tune in to your body. Every individual is unique, especially when it comes to fitness levels and physical conditions. Throughout this week, pay attention to how your body responds to various movements. It's normal to feel some initial stiffness or fatigue, but you should never feel sharp pain. If you do, stop immediately and consult with a healthcare professional.

Setting the Stage for Success

Create Your Exercise Space:
Designate a safe, comfortable area in your home for your workouts. Ideally, you'll need a sturdy chair, a yoga mat or a soft carpet, light weights (1-5 pounds), and water for hydration. Ensure that there are no tripping hazards around your workout area to keep yourself safe.

Gather Your Equipment:

Chair: A strong, armless chair with a flat seat. It should be stable and provide good support for seated exercises.
Weights: If you don't have dumbbells, you can use household items like water bottles or bags of rice. Start light; you can increase the weight as you get stronger.
Comfortable Clothing: Wear breathable, loose-fitting clothes that allow you to move freely. A good pair of supportive shoes will also help.
Daily Exercise Routine
Frequency: Aim to exercise 5 days a week, allowing for two rest days. This routine will include a combination of chair yoga, strength training, and light stretching.

Duration: Each session should last about 20-30 minutes, which is manageable and effective for easing into a routine.

Monday: Chair Yoga Session
Warm-Up (5 minutes):

Start by sitting tall in your chair.
Take a few deep breaths, inhaling through your nose and exhaling through your mouth.
Perform gentle neck rolls, then shoulder rolls to release tension.
Main Sequence (15 minutes):

Seated Cat-Cow Stretch:

Inhale as you arch your back and look up (cow pose).
Exhale as you round your back and tuck your chin (cat pose).
Repeat for 5 cycles.
Seated Forward Bend:

With feet flat on the floor, inhale and raise your arms overhead.
Exhale and hinge at the hips, reaching your hands toward your feet.
Hold for 5 deep breaths.
Gentle Chair Twist:

Inhale as you lengthen your spine.
Exhale and twist to the right, placing your left hand on your right knee and right hand on the chair.
Hold for 5 breaths, then switch sides.
Seated Mountain Pose:

Sit tall with feet flat, arms by your sides.
Inhale and raise your arms overhead, palms facing each other.
Hold for 5 breaths, focusing on your posture.
Cool Down (5 minutes):

Repeat deep breathing exercises, closing your eyes and visualizing your body relaxing.
Tuesday: Upper Body Strength Training
Warm-Up (5 minutes):

Perform gentle shoulder rolls and wrist circles.
Main Routine (20 minutes):

Seated Bicep Curls:

Sit up straight and hold a weight in each hand.
Curl the weights toward your shoulders, then lower them back down.
Perform 10-15 repetitions.
Seated Overhead Press:

Hold weights at shoulder height.
Press weights overhead, then lower back to shoulders.
Perform 10-15 repetitions.
Chair-Assisted Lateral Raise:

Hold weights at your sides, and raise them to shoulder height.
Control the weights back down.
Perform 10-15 repetitions.
Seated Row:

Using a resistance band, anchor it under your chair, and pull the band towards you as you squeeze your shoulder blades together.
Perform 10-15 repetitions.
Cool Down (5 minutes):

Stretch your arms and shoulders, holding each stretch for 15-20 seconds.
Wednesday: Lower Body Strength Training
Warm-Up (5 minutes):

March in place to get your blood flowing.
Main Routine (20 minutes):

Seated Leg Lifts:

Sit tall and extend one leg straight out.
Hold for a few seconds, then lower it back down.
Alternate legs for 10 repetitions each.
Chair-Assisted Squats:

Stand in front of the chair, lower your body as if sitting down, then return to standing.
Perform 10-15 repetitions.
Seated Side Leg Raises:

While seated, lift your leg to the side.
Hold briefly and lower. Alternate legs for 10 repetitions each.
Calf Raises:

Stand behind the chair for support.
Rise onto your toes, then lower back down.
Perform 10-15 repetitions.
Cool Down (5 minutes):

Stretch your legs and hips, focusing on hamstrings and quadriceps.
Thursday: Chair Yoga Session (Repeat Monday's Routine)
This session can help reinforce the techniques learned earlier in the week, allowing you to refine your movements.

Friday: Full Body Stretch and Light Cardio
Warm-Up (5 minutes):

March in place or walk around your space to get your heart rate up.
Main Routine (20 minutes):

Seated Forward Bend: (As before)

Seated Side Stretch:

While seated, reach one arm overhead and lean to the opposite side.
Hold for 5 breaths, then switch sides.
Torso Twist:

Sit up tall and rotate your torso to one side, using your arm for support.
Hold for 5 breaths, then switch sides.
Gentle Marching:

Stand and march in place for 5-10 minutes to get the heart rate up.
Cool Down (5 minutes):

Deep breathing while seated or lying down to relax.
Monitoring Progress and Staying Motivated
During this first week, it's essential to keep track of your feelings, progress, and any challenges you encounter. Use a journal to note how you felt before and after each workout, any improvements you noticed in your flexibility or strength, and any adjustments you may want to make in the following weeks.

Stay Motivated:

Set small, achievable goals. Celebrate completing each day's workout!
Consider enlisting a friend or family member to join you in these exercises. Working out with someone can be encouraging and enjoyable.

By the end of Week 1, you should feel more comfortable with your body's movements and may notice an increase in your energy levels. Remember, this week is just the beginning. As you progress, you'll gain strength, flexibility, and confidence, paving the way for the subsequent weeks of your exercise plan. Stay committed, and enjoy the journey toward a healthier, more active life!

Week 2: Increasing Strength and Flexibility

Welcome to Week 2 of your journey to a healthier, more active lifestyle! Now that you've established a foundation in Week 1, it's time to build on those skills by increasing both your strength and flexibility. This week's focus is on gradual progression, allowing you to enhance your physical abilities while ensuring you remain comfortable and safe.

Understanding Strength and Flexibility

Before diving into the specifics of your workout plan, let's take a moment to understand the importance of strength and flexibility, particularly as we age.

Strength is not just about lifting heavy weights; it's about functional fitness. Functional strength allows you to perform daily activities, such as lifting groceries, getting up from a chair, and maintaining your balance. It contributes significantly to your overall health, improving your metabolism and helping with weight management.

Flexibility, on the other hand, refers to the range of motion in your joints. Good flexibility enhances your ability to move freely, reduces the risk of injuries, and alleviates discomfort in your muscles and joints. This week's routine will incorporate exercises designed to enhance both of these essential fitness components.

Weekly Structure

Your exercise plan this week will consist of five workout days that blend chair yoga and strength training, allowing your body to adapt and grow stronger without overwhelming it. Aim to include at least two rest days, which can also include light activity such as walking or gentle stretching.

Weekly Overview:

- - Day 1: Chair Yoga for Flexibility
- - Day 2: Upper Body Strength Training
- - Day 3: Active Recovery and Stretching
- - Day 4: Lower Body Strength Training
- - Day 5: Full Body Strength and Flexibility Routine
- - Day 6: Rest or Light Activity
- - Day 7: Reflect and Prepare for Week 3

Day 1: Chair Yoga for Flexibility

Goal: Enhance your flexibility and increase relaxation.

Warm-Up (5 minutes):
- Seated Cat-Cow Stretch: While sitting, arch your back (cat) and then curve it gently (cow). Repeat 5 times.

- Neck Rolls: Slowly roll your neck in a circular motion, both directions (5 times each).

Chair Yoga Sequence (20 minutes):

1. Seated Forward Bend (Hold for 30 seconds):
   Sit tall and hinge at your hips to reach towards your toes. Feel the stretch in your lower back and hamstrings.

2. Gentle Chair Twist (Hold for 30 seconds each side):
   Sit with a straight back, place your right hand on the back of the chair, and twist to the right, keeping your hips facing forward. Repeat on the left side.

3. Seated Side Stretch (Hold for 30 seconds each side):
   Raise your right arm overhead and lean to the left, feeling the stretch along your side. Switch sides.

4. Seated Pigeon Pose (Hold for 30 seconds each side):
   Place your right ankle on your left knee, sitting up tall. Lean forward gently to deepen the stretch.

5. Seated Mountain Pose (Hold for 1 minute):
   Sit tall with feet flat on the ground, arms by your sides. Take deep breaths, focusing on grounding yourself.

Cool Down (5 minutes):
- Deep Breathing: Inhale deeply through your nose and exhale slowly through your mouth, allowing your body to relax completely.

Day 2: Upper Body Strength Training

Goal: Build upper body strength and improve muscle tone.

Warm-Up (5 minutes):
- Arm Circles: Extend your arms out to the side and make small circles, gradually increasing the size (1 minute each direction).
- Shoulder Rolls: Roll your shoulders forward and backward (10 times each).

Strength Exercises (20 minutes):

1. Seated Bicep Curls (3 sets of 10-12 reps):

Sit up straight and hold light weights in both hands. Curl the weights towards your shoulders, keeping your elbows close to your body.

2. Chair-Assisted Overhead Press (3 sets of 10-12 reps):
With weights at shoulder height, press upward, extending your arms fully overhead. Lower back to the start position.

3. Seated Lateral Raises (3 sets of 10-12 reps):
With weights at your sides, lift your arms out to the sides to shoulder height, then lower back down.

4. Seated Row (3 sets of 10-12 reps):
Hold weights in front of you, elbows bent. Pull weights towards your chest, squeezing your shoulder blades together.

5. Chair-Assisted Tricep Extensions (3 sets of 10-12 reps):
Raise a weight overhead with both hands. Lower it behind your head while keeping your elbows close, then return to the starting position.

Cool Down (5 minutes):
- Upper Body Stretch: Extend your arms overhead and lean to each side. Hold each side for 30 seconds.

Day 3: Active Recovery and Stretching

Goal: Allow your muscles to recover while promoting flexibility.

Light Activity (20 minutes):
- Take a leisurely walk, focusing on your breath and posture. Aim for a comfortable pace that encourages movement without strain.

Stretching Routine (15 minutes):

1. Neck Stretch:
Gently tilt your head to one side, using your hand to deepen the stretch (30 seconds each side).

2. Shoulder Stretch:
Bring one arm across your body and gently pull it closer with the opposite arm (30 seconds each side).

3. Wrist Stretch:
   Extend one arm forward, palm facing up, and gently pull back on the fingers with the opposite hand (30 seconds each side).

4. Hip Flexor Stretch:
   While seated, extend one leg out and lean forward gently, feeling the stretch in your hip (30 seconds each side).

Cool Down:
- Deep Breathing: Focus on your breath to relax.

Day 4: Lower Body Strength Training

Goal: Enhance lower body strength and stability.

Warm-Up (5 minutes):
- Seated Leg Extensions: While sitting, extend one leg at a time (10 reps each leg).
- Ankle Rolls: Rotate your ankles in circles, both directions (1 minute each).

Strength Exercises (20 minutes):

1. Chair-Assisted Squats (3 sets of 10-12 reps):
   Stand in front of the chair, lower yourself down as if sitting, then rise back up without fully sitting.

2. Seated Leg Lifts (3 sets of 10-12 reps per leg):
   Sit tall and extend one leg out in front of you, keeping it straight. Hold for a moment before lowering.

3. Chair-Assisted Calf Raises (3 sets of 10-12 reps):
   Hold onto the chair for support. Rise onto your toes, then lower back down.

4. Side Leg Raises (3 sets of 10-12 reps per leg):
   Stand beside the chair and lift your leg out to the side, keeping it straight. Lower back down.

5. Chair Glute Squeeze (3 sets of 10-12 reps):
   Sit tall and squeeze your glutes together, holding for a few seconds before releasing.

Cool Down (5 minutes):

- Lower Body Stretch: Stretch your hamstrings, quadriceps, and calves, holding each stretch for 30 seconds.

Day 5: Full Body Strength and Flexibility Routine

Goal: Integrate strength and flexibility exercises for a comprehensive workout.

Warm-Up (5 minutes):
- March in Place: Gently march in place, lifting your knees slightly and swinging your arms.

Full Body Circuit (30 minutes):

1. Chair Yoga Flow (5 minutes):
   Combine seated forward bends, gentle twists, and stretches to warm up.

2. Upper Body Circuit (15 minutes):
   Repeat the upper body strength exercises from Day 2 but reduce the rest time between sets to keep your heart rate up.

3. Lower Body Circuit (10 minutes):
   Repeat the lower body exercises from Day 4, maintaining good form and controlled movements.

Cool Down (5 minutes):
- Full Body Stretching Routine: Focus on all major muscle groups, holding each stretch for 30 seconds.

Day 6: Rest or Light Activity

Listen to your body and take this day for rest or light activity. This could include:

- Gentle Walking: Enjoy a stroll in your neighborhood or a local park.
- Chair Yoga: Engage in a few gentle chair yoga poses for relaxation.
- Social Activities: Consider inviting friends for a gentle walk or a yoga session at home.

Day 7: Reflect and Prepare for Week 3

This day is not just about rest; it's a time for reflection and preparation. Take some time to journal about your experiences over the past week. Ask yourself:

- How did my body feel during exercises?
- What improvements have I noticed in my strength or flexibility?
- Did I face any challenges? How can I address them moving forward?
- What goals do I want to set for next week?

This reflection will help you stay motivated and committed to your fitness journey. As you prepare for Week 3, think about any new goals you want to set, perhaps focusing on increasing your repetitions or exploring

Week 3: Building Endurance and Weight Loss

Welcome to Week 3 of your exercise journey! By now, you've built a solid foundation with chair yoga and strength training exercises. In this week, we will focus on enhancing your endurance and accelerating weight loss. This chapter will guide you through a comprehensive plan that not only increases your physical capabilities but also reinforces your commitment to a healthier lifestyle.

Understanding Endurance and Its Importance
Endurance refers to the ability of your body to sustain prolonged exercise. It's not just about stamina; it encompasses both cardiovascular endurance and muscular endurance. Improving your endurance will enable you to engage in daily activities with more ease and less fatigue, contributing significantly to your overall quality of life.

For seniors, enhancing endurance is crucial. It can help reduce the risk of falls, enhance mobility, and improve cardiovascular health. This week, we'll incorporate exercises that elevate your heart rate, strengthen your muscles, and promote weight loss by increasing your caloric expenditure.

Weekly Exercise Schedule
Daily Schedule Overview:

- Day 1: Chair Yoga for Flexibility and Core Strength
- Day 2: Upper Body Strength and Cardio Intervals
- Day 3: Lower Body Strength and Stability
- Day 4: Active Recovery with Gentle Movement
- Day 5: Full-Body Circuit Workout
- Day 6: Chair Yoga Flow and Relaxation
- Day 7: Review, Reflect, and Prepare for Week 4

Note: Each workout should begin with a warm-up and end with a cool-down. This ensures you're prepared for the exercises and helps to prevent injury.

Day 1: Chair Yoga for Flexibility and Core Strength
Duration: 30 minutes

Warm-Up (5 minutes):

Neck Rolls: Gently roll your head in circles to loosen the neck.
Shoulder Shrugs: Raise your shoulders toward your ears and release.
Chair Yoga Poses (20 minutes):

Seated Cat-Cow Stretch (5 reps): Helps improve spinal flexibility.
Seated Forward Bend (30 seconds): Stretches the lower back.
Seated Side Stretch (30 seconds per side): Opens up the ribcage and improves breathing.
Seated Twist (30 seconds per side): Enhances spinal mobility and digestion.
Seated Mountain Pose (1 minute): Focus on breathing and grounding yourself.
Core Engagement:

Seated Leg Lifts (3 sets of 10 reps per leg): Strengthens the core and hip flexors.
Cool Down (5 minutes):

Gentle breathing and meditation to center your mind and body.
Day 2: Upper Body Strength and Cardio Intervals
Duration: 30-40 minutes

Warm-Up (5 minutes):

Arm Circles and Wrist Rotations.
Strength Exercises (20 minutes):

Bicep Curls with Light Weights (3 sets of 10 reps): For arm strength.
Chair-Assisted Push-Ups (3 sets of 5-10 reps): Enhances upper body strength.
Seated Overhead Press (3 sets of 10 reps): Focuses on shoulders and triceps.
Chest Squeeze with a Pillow (3 sets of 10 reps): Works the chest muscles.
Cardio Intervals (10 minutes):

Alternate 1 minute of seated marching with 30 seconds of seated punches.
Repeat this sequence for 10 minutes to elevate your heart rate.
Cool Down (5 minutes):

Gentle stretches focusing on the arms and shoulders.
Day 3: Lower Body Strength and Stability
Duration: 30-40 minutes

Warm-Up (5 minutes):

Ankle Rolls and Knee Lifts.
Strength Exercises (20 minutes):

Seated Leg Extensions (3 sets of 10 reps per leg): Strengthens the quadriceps.
Chair-Assisted Squats (3 sets of 10 reps): Engages the entire lower body.
Seated Side Leg Raises (3 sets of 10 reps per leg): Works the hips and outer thighs.
Calf Raises (3 sets of 10 reps): Improves ankle stability and leg strength.
Stability Work (10 minutes):

One-Leg Stand (30 seconds per leg, 3 sets): Enhances balance and coordination.
Practice standing tall and engaging your core.
Cool Down (5 minutes):

Stretch your legs and lower back to promote flexibility.
Day 4: Active Recovery with Gentle Movement
Duration: 20-30 minutes

Engage in gentle activities such as walking around your home or yard, or practicing slow chair yoga. Focus on relaxation and breathing. This day is vital for recovery, allowing your muscles to heal while maintaining light activity to keep your body engaged.

Day 5: Full-Body Circuit Workout
Duration: 40-50 minutes

Warm-Up (5 minutes):

Gentle movements to get your heart rate up.
Circuit Exercises (30 minutes):

Perform each exercise for 1 minute, then rest for 30 seconds before moving to the next:
Seated Marching
Seated Bicep Curls
Chair Squats
Seated Side Leg Raises
Seated Overhead Press
Repeat the circuit twice.
Cool Down (5-10 minutes):

Focus on slow, deep breathing and gentle stretches for the entire body.
Day 6: Chair Yoga Flow and Relaxation
Duration: 30 minutes

Engage in a gentle chair yoga flow that incorporates the poses you've learned over the past weeks. Focus on the connection between your breath and movements. Use this session to reflect on your progress, appreciating how far you've come in just three weeks.

Warm-Up (5 minutes):

Deep Breaths and Gentle Neck Stretches.
Chair Yoga Flow (20 minutes):

Incorporate multiple poses into a flowing sequence.
Allow for transitions between poses to keep your body moving fluidly.
Cool Down (5 minutes):

Spend this time in a comfortable seated position, focusing on your breath and allowing your body to relax completely.
Day 7: Review, Reflect, and Prepare for Week 4
Take time today to assess your progress. Reflect on how you feel physically and mentally. Consider keeping a journal to track your experiences, challenges, and triumphs. This practice can motivate you as you move into the next week.

Goals Check: Have you noticed improvements in your endurance and flexibility?

What Worked: Identify which exercises you enjoyed the most and felt beneficial.

What to Improve: Note any exercises that were too challenging or caused discomfort.

Nutrition and Hydration

To support your exercise routine, ensure you're staying hydrated throughout the week. Water plays a crucial role in muscle recovery and overall health. Aim for at least 8 cups a day, adjusting based on your activity level.

In addition, focus on nutrient-rich foods that support weight loss and energy levels. Incorporate lean proteins, whole grains, healthy fats, and plenty of fruits and vegetables into your meals. This balanced approach will enhance your results and help you feel your best.

By the end of Week 3, you should begin to notice significant improvements in your endurance and flexibility. Your body will adapt to the increased activity, and you may find yourself feeling more energetic and less fatigued. Remember, consistency is key. As you prepare for Week 4, keep your goals in mind and look forward to the continued journey of health and wellness. Together, we're building a healthier, stronger you!

Week 4: Maintaining Your Progress

Congratulations! You've made it to Week 4 of your exercise plan. By now, you've taken significant strides toward enhancing your strength, flexibility, and overall well-being through chair yoga and strength training. This week is all about maintaining your hard-earned progress and building upon the foundation you've established. Remember, the goal isn't just about weight loss or flexibility; it's about creating a sustainable lifestyle that empowers you for the long haul.

Understanding the Importance of Maintenance

After three weeks of commitment to your fitness journey, it's crucial to understand the importance of maintenance. Many people often think of fitness as a short-term goal: lose weight, tone muscles, or become more flexible. However, true wellness involves a long-term approach, where you incorporate healthy habits into your daily routine.

Why Maintenance Matters: Your body has adapted to the exercises you've been performing, and it craves variety and progression. Maintenance is not just about keeping your progress but enhancing it and preventing plateaus that can lead to frustration and demotivation.

Psychological Benefits: Regular exercise releases endorphins, the "feel-good" hormones that can significantly boost your mood. By continuing your routine, you'll not only maintain your physical results but also support your mental health.

Building Habits: Consistency is key. By dedicating time to exercise this week, you solidify your habits, making it easier to continue your fitness journey in the future.

Maintaining Your Routine
As we dive into Week 4, let's focus on how to maintain and even elevate your fitness levels with a mix of chair yoga, strength training, and mindful eating.

1. Chair Yoga Flow: Daily Practice
Daily Chair Yoga Routine
Incorporating daily chair yoga can enhance flexibility, improve posture, and reduce stress. Aim for 15-20 minutes each day. Here's a simple flow to follow:

Seated Cat-Cow Stretch (2 minutes): Start in a seated position. Inhale as you arch your back and look up (cow), then exhale as you round your back and tuck your chin (cat). Repeat for one minute.

Seated Forward Bend (2 minutes): With feet flat on the floor, hinge at your hips to fold forward, reaching towards the floor or your ankles. Hold for several breaths.

Seated Twist (3 minutes): Place your right hand on the back of your chair and twist to the right, using your left hand to deepen the stretch. Hold for five breaths, then switch sides.

Side Stretch (2 minutes): Raise your right arm overhead and lean to the left. Hold for five breaths, feeling the stretch along your side. Switch sides.

Neck Stretch (2 minutes): Gently tilt your head to one side, bringing your ear toward your shoulder. Hold for five breaths and switch sides.

Seated Mountain Pose (3 minutes): Sit tall, shoulders relaxed, palms on your thighs. Focus on your breath, visualizing yourself grounded and strong.

Benefits of Chair Yoga: Each of these poses not only helps maintain flexibility but also promotes relaxation, which is vital as you progress.

2. Strength Training Routine: Consistency and Variety
Weekly Strength Training Plan
This week, we'll maintain your strength with slightly increased intensity. Here's a balanced routine you can perform three times this week, ensuring a day of rest in between.

Day 1: Upper Body Focus

Seated Bicep Curls (3 sets of 10-15 reps): Use light weights. Sit upright and curl the weights towards your shoulders, keeping your elbows close to your body.

Seated Shoulder Press (3 sets of 10-15 reps): Press weights overhead, focusing on engaging your core.

Chair-Assisted Tricep Extensions (3 sets of 10-15 reps): Hold a weight in both hands above your head, lower it behind your head, and press it back up.

Seated Row with Resistance Band (3 sets of 10-15 reps): Secure a resistance band at your feet and pull towards you, squeezing your shoulder blades together.

Day 2: Lower Body Focus

Seated Leg Lifts (3 sets of 10-15 reps each leg): Extend one leg at a time, holding at the top for a moment before lowering.

Chair-Assisted Squats (3 sets of 10-15 reps): Stand in front of the chair, lower your body as if sitting down, and return to standing.

Calf Raises (3 sets of 10-15 reps): Stand behind the chair and lift your heels off the ground, balancing on your toes.

Day 3: Full Body Integration

Seated Marching (3 sets of 1 minute): Lift knees alternately, engaging your core as if marching in place.

Side Leg Raises (3 sets of 10-15 reps): While seated, lift your leg out to the side and lower it back down. Switch sides.

Chair-Assisted Deadlifts (3 sets of 10-15 reps): Stand and hinge at the hips while holding onto the chair for balance, then return to standing.

Variety is Key: This week, feel free to add resistance or increase repetitions as you feel comfortable. Keeping your muscles guessing is essential to continued improvement.

3. Mindful Eating for Sustainable Progress

As you maintain your physical activities, it's crucial to support your efforts with mindful eating. Nutrition plays a significant role in your ability to perform and recover from exercises.

Balanced Meals: Ensure each meal consists of protein, healthy fats, and complex carbohydrates. Think grilled chicken or fish, a variety of vegetables, whole grains, and healthy oils.

Hydration: Drink plenty of water throughout the day, especially before and after your workouts. Staying hydrated enhances performance and aids in recovery.

Portion Control: Listen to your body's hunger cues. Eating slowly and mindfully helps you recognize when you're satisfied, preventing overeating.

Healthy Snacks: Opt for nutrient-dense snacks like Greek yogurt with berries, nuts, or hummus with veggies to keep your energy levels stable.

4. Track Your Progress

Maintaining progress also involves keeping an eye on your improvements. Consider the following:

Fitness Journal: Document your workouts, noting the exercises, sets, reps, and how you felt during each session. This reflection will help you recognize growth and areas needing adjustment.

Flexibility Assessments: At the end of the week, test your flexibility with simple stretches. Notice any improvements in your range of motion or ease of movement.

Celebrate Small Wins: Recognize and celebrate every small achievement, whether it's completing a workout, increasing weights, or feeling more energetic.

5. Stay Motivated

Finally, motivation is essential to maintaining progress. Here are some strategies:

Buddy System: Consider inviting a friend or family member to join you in your routines. Having a workout partner can enhance accountability and make exercising more enjoyable.

Set New Goals: As you maintain your current fitness level, think about new challenges. Perhaps aim to increase your strength training weights or try a new chair yoga pose.

Reward Yourself: Treat yourself when you achieve specific goals. It could be a new workout outfit, a massage, or even a special outing—whatever makes you feel appreciated for your efforts.

Week 4 is a pivotal time in your fitness journey. As you maintain your progress, remember that fitness is a lifelong commitment. Each step you take, no matter how small, contributes to your overall health and happiness. You've built a foundation of strength and flexibility; now, it's about cultivating these practices into your daily life. With dedication and mindfulness, you can continue to thrive well beyond these four weeks. Embrace this journey, and remember: every bit of effort counts toward a healthier, more vibrant you.

How to Track Your Success: Weight, Flexibility, and Strength Gains

Tracking your progress is essential for maintaining motivation and achieving your fitness goals, especially as a senior engaging in chair yoga and strength training. This detailed guide will provide you with practical methods and insights into effectively measuring weight loss, flexibility, and strength gains. Understanding these metrics not only helps you see how far you've come but also allows you to adjust your routine for optimal results.

Why Tracking Matters
Before diving into specific methods, it's important to understand why tracking your progress is crucial:

Motivation: Seeing tangible results can be incredibly motivating. Whether it's losing a few pounds, being able to reach your toes, or lifting heavier weights, these achievements can inspire you to keep going.

Accountability: When you have a record of your workouts, meals, and physical changes, it holds you accountable to yourself. You're less likely to skip workouts or stray from your diet if you know you'll be tracking your progress.

Adjustment: Tracking allows you to identify patterns and make adjustments to your routine as needed. If something isn't working, you'll know to change it.

Celebration: Every small win deserves recognition. Tracking your success allows you to celebrate milestones, no matter how small, which boosts your confidence and encourages continued effort.

Tracking Weight Loss
1. Weigh Yourself Regularly

To effectively track weight loss:

Frequency: Weigh yourself once a week, ideally at the same time of day and under the same conditions (e.g., after waking up and using the bathroom). This consistency will provide the most accurate representation of your weight trend over time.

Scale Accuracy: Ensure your scale is on a flat, hard surface and is properly calibrated. A reliable scale will give you more accurate readings.

Mind the Fluctuations: Understand that weight can fluctuate daily due to various factors, including hydration, diet, and even muscle gain. Focus on the overall trend rather than daily changes.

2. Record Your Weight

Keep a dedicated journal or use a digital app to log your weight each week. Create a simple chart or spreadsheet to visualize your weight loss journey. You can also include notes about your diet, exercise, and how you felt that week, as these factors contribute to your weight changes.

3. Set Realistic Goals

When tracking weight loss, it's important to set achievable goals. Instead of aiming for drastic weight loss, focus on gradual changes—1 to 2 pounds per week is a healthy target. Setting short-term goals, such as losing 5% of your current weight, can also provide motivation and make the process feel more attainable.

Measuring Flexibility Gains
1. Flexibility Tests

Tracking flexibility can be done through specific tests that measure the range of motion in your joints. Here are a few methods:

Sit-and-Reach Test: Sit on the floor with your legs extended straight in front of you. Reach forward as far as possible while keeping your knees straight. Measure the distance between your fingertips and your toes. Track your progress every few weeks.

Shoulder Flexibility Test: Stand or sit comfortably and reach one arm over your shoulder and down your back while reaching the other arm up your back. Measure how far you can go. This test is particularly useful for assessing shoulder flexibility, which can be crucial for daily activities.

Hip Flexibility Test: Stand up straight and lift one knee to your chest, holding it there for a few seconds. Alternate legs and track how high you can lift your knee. The higher you can lift, the more flexible your hips are becoming.

2. Document Your Progress

Keep a flexibility log in the same journal where you track your weight. Write down the results of each flexibility test, noting any improvements over time. Use a ruler or measuring tape for precise measurements, and consider taking photos or videos of your stretches to visually compare your progress.

3. Regular Stretching Routine

Incorporate a regular stretching routine into your workouts. Consistency is key for improving flexibility. Consider dedicating 10–15 minutes before or after your chair yoga and strength training sessions to focus on stretching major muscle groups.

Tracking Strength Gains
1. Strength Assessment

To track strength gains, perform a few simple strength assessments at regular intervals (e.g., every 4–6 weeks):

Chair Stand Test: Sit in a chair and stand up without using your hands. Count how many times you can do this in 30 seconds. Track how the number improves over time.

Bicep Curl Test: Using light weights (1-5 pounds), perform bicep curls. Track the number of repetitions you can complete in one set. Gradually increase the weight and repetitions to assess progress.

Wall Push-Up Test: Stand about an arm's length from a wall, place your palms on the wall, and perform push-ups. Track how many you can do in one minute, and aim to increase this number over time.

2. Record Your Exercises

Keep a strength training log where you note the exercises performed, weights used, repetitions, and sets. This log will help you visualize your progress and encourage you to lift heavier weights or complete more repetitions as you gain strength.

3. Focus on Progression

Once you feel comfortable with a certain weight or number of repetitions, aim to gradually increase the difficulty. This can be achieved by:

Increasing Weight: Add small increments of weight (e.g., 1–2 pounds) to your routine every couple of weeks.

Increasing Repetitions: Once you can comfortably perform the desired repetitions, add a few more to your sets.

Adding Variations: Incorporate new exercises that challenge your muscles differently. For instance, if you're comfortable with seated bicep curls, try standing curls or tricep extensions.

Combining Metrics for Overall Progress
While tracking weight, flexibility, and strength gains separately is valuable, consider integrating these metrics for a comprehensive view of your fitness journey:

Create a Weekly Dashboard: Combine your weight, flexibility test results, and strength assessment into a single weekly dashboard. This overview allows you to see how improvements in one area may correlate with changes in others.

Visual Representations: Use charts and graphs to visualize your progress. Many apps offer graphical representations of weight loss, which can be motivating.

Reflect on Your Journey: Take time each month to reflect on your progress. Consider journaling about how you feel physically and emotionally. Celebrate your achievements, no matter how small.

The Emotional Aspect of Tracking
It's essential to acknowledge the emotional component of tracking your progress. As you observe changes in your body and abilities, take note of your feelings:

Self-Esteem: Achievements in weight loss, flexibility, and strength can significantly boost your self-esteem. Recognizing these accomplishments can encourage you to continue striving for more.

Mindfulness: The process of tracking your progress encourages mindfulness. You become more aware of your body's abilities and limitations, leading to a more holistic understanding of your health.

Community and Support: Share your progress with friends, family, or exercise groups. Having a support system can enhance accountability and motivation.

Tracking your success in weight, flexibility, and strength gains is not merely about numbers; it's about understanding your body, setting realistic goals, and celebrating your achievements. By implementing effective tracking methods and reflecting on your progress, you'll not only stay motivated but also cultivate a positive mindset toward your fitness journey. Remember, every small step counts, and the journey to better health and fitness is one worth celebrating. Embrace the process, enjoy the workouts, and take pride in the progress you make along the way.

How to Make Exercise a Daily Habit

Establishing a regular exercise routine can feel daunting, especially as we age. However, creating a daily exercise habit is not only beneficial; it's transformative. For seniors over 60, regular physical activity enhances mobility, promotes weight loss, strengthens muscles, and significantly improves overall well-being. So, how do you transition from occasional exercise to a consistent, fulfilling routine? Let's explore some effective strategies to make exercise an integral part of your daily life.

Understanding the Importance of Habit Formation
1. The Science of Habits
Habits are formed through repetition and consistency. When you perform an action regularly, it becomes automatic—part of your daily routine. The key is to associate exercise with positive experiences. By understanding how habits work, you can create a framework that encourages consistency. Research shows that it takes an average of 66 days to establish a new habit, so patience is essential.

2. Start with "Why"
Understanding your motivation is crucial. Ask yourself:

Why do you want to exercise?
Is it to lose weight, gain strength, improve flexibility, or enhance your quality of life?

What personal goals do you want to achieve?

Clarifying your "why" creates a powerful internal drive. Write down your reasons and keep them somewhere visible to remind yourself of your goals.

Creating a Sustainable Routine

1. Set Realistic Goals

Begin with achievable, specific goals. Rather than saying, "I want to exercise more," aim for something concrete like, "I will do chair yoga for 20 minutes every morning." This clarity transforms your intention into actionable steps.

2. Design Your Weekly Schedule

Consistency thrives on structure. Consider designing a weekly exercise schedule. Allocate specific days and times for your workouts, just as you would for any other important appointment. Incorporate variety to keep it interesting—mix chair yoga, strength training, and stretching exercises throughout the week.

3. Find Activities You Enjoy

Exercise doesn't have to be a chore. Explore different types of physical activities to find what you enjoy the most. You might love chair yoga, walking in nature, dancing, or even gardening. Enjoyment is key to maintaining motivation. When you look forward to your workout, it becomes less of a task and more of a pleasure.

Making Exercise Convenient

1. Create an Exercise Space

Designate a specific area in your home for exercise. Ensure it's well-lit, free of distractions, and equipped with everything you need (weights, mat, chair). Having a dedicated space makes it easier to jump into your routine without the hassle of setting up.

2. Keep Equipment Accessible

Store your exercise equipment in a location where it's easily accessible. If your weights are in the garage or basement, you might be less inclined to use them. Consider keeping light weights or resistance bands near your chair or in the living room.

3. Pair Exercise with Daily Activities

Integrating exercise into your daily routine can help make it habitual. For instance, you might do chair exercises while watching TV, practice deep breathing and stretches while reading, or take short walks after meals. This not only reinforces your exercise habit but also makes it feel less daunting.

Building a Support System

1. Involve Family and Friends
Engaging loved ones can significantly boost motivation. Invite family members or friends to join you in your workouts. Sharing the experience makes it more enjoyable and fosters a sense of accountability.

2. Join a Class or Group
Consider joining a community exercise class, such as chair yoga or a senior fitness group. These classes provide social interaction, structured guidance, and encouragement. Being part of a community can motivate you to stay consistent.

3. Use Technology to Your Advantage
In today's digital age, there are countless resources at your fingertips. Use fitness apps, online videos, or DVDs tailored to seniors to guide your workouts. These tools can provide variety and help you stay engaged with your routine.

Overcoming Barriers
1. Acknowledge Challenges
Life can be unpredictable, and barriers to exercise may arise—be it fatigue, illness, or scheduling conflicts. Acknowledge these challenges without judgment. Understanding that obstacles are a part of the journey allows you to adjust your plans rather than give up.

2. Listen to Your Body
It's essential to be attuned to your body's signals. If you're feeling particularly tired or unwell, it's okay to modify your workout or take a rest day. Consistency is important, but so is your overall health and well-being. Always consult with your healthcare provider when starting a new exercise program or if you experience any concerning symptoms.

3. Celebrate Small Wins
Celebrate every step of your journey. Whether it's completing a week of workouts, mastering a new exercise, or simply feeling more energetic, acknowledging your progress reinforces positive feelings around exercise. Keep a journal to track your workouts and reflect on how you feel, both physically and emotionally.

Staying Motivated for the Long Haul
1. Create a Reward System
Incorporate a reward system to keep you motivated. After reaching specific milestones—be it a week of consistent exercise or a weight loss goal—treat yourself to something you enjoy, like a massage, a new book, or a day out with friends.

2. Refresh Your Routine Regularly

To prevent boredom, change your routine every few weeks. Explore new exercises, vary your schedule, or join a different class. The novelty can reignite your passion and commitment to staying active.

3. Maintain a Positive Mindset
A positive attitude toward exercise can significantly impact your willingness to commit. Focus on the benefits you experience, such as increased energy, improved mood, and greater flexibility. Surround yourself with positivity, whether through uplifting quotes, supportive friends, or motivational content.

4. Reflect on Your Journey
Regularly take time to reflect on your fitness journey. Consider the challenges you've overcome, the successes you've achieved, and how far you've come. This reflection can reinforce your commitment and inspire you to keep moving forward.

Incorporating exercise into your daily routine is a journey, not a sprint. As you embark on this path, remember that every small step counts. By understanding your motivations, creating a sustainable routine, finding enjoyment in your workouts, and building a supportive community, you can establish a lasting exercise habit. Embrace the process, celebrate your progress, and recognize that maintaining an active lifestyle is one of the most empowering choices you can make for your health and well-being. Your journey toward fitness is not just about physical changes; it's about enhancing your quality of life and embracing the vitality that comes with staying active. You've got this!

Staying Connected: Encouraging Friends or Family to Join You

As we embark on the journey of fitness, especially after the age of 60, one crucial aspect often overlooked is the power of connection. Engaging friends or family members in your fitness journey can significantly enhance your experience, motivation, and overall results. It's not just about exercising; it's about building a community of support that makes the process enjoyable and sustainable.

The Importance of Social Connections in Fitness
Motivation and Accountability: Exercising with others can provide the motivation needed to stick to your routine. When you have a workout buddy, you're more likely to stay committed. The accountability of knowing someone else is counting on you can make all the difference on those days when you feel like skipping your workout. A simple text or call to your friend or

family member can be the push you need to lace up those sneakers and hit the mat or chair for some yoga.

Shared Experiences: Working out together creates shared experiences that foster deeper relationships. Whether it's laughing at each other while trying a new stretch or celebrating small victories, these moments build camaraderie. Shared experiences enhance the joy of exercise, transforming it from a solitary chore into a fun and interactive activity.

Emotional Support: Fitness can be an emotional journey, especially when you're facing challenges such as weight loss, physical limitations, or motivation hurdles. Having friends or family members alongside you offers emotional support, making it easier to navigate these ups and downs. You can share your struggles, encourage each other, and celebrate milestones together, creating a positive atmosphere.

Healthy Competition: Engaging in friendly competition can also be a fantastic way to motivate each other. Setting small challenges, such as who can hold a pose the longest or who can complete more repetitions of an exercise, adds an element of fun and excitement to your routine. Just be sure that the competition remains light-hearted; the goal is to uplift each other, not create unnecessary pressure.

Learning and Sharing Knowledge: Working out with others can also be an educational experience. Sharing techniques, tips, and tricks can enhance everyone's understanding of the exercises and promote better form and effectiveness. Perhaps a family member has experience with yoga or strength training; they can share insights or lead sessions, enriching the group's knowledge base.

How to Encourage Friends or Family to Join You
Now that we understand the importance of connection, let's explore some effective strategies for encouraging friends or family members to join your fitness journey.

Start with an Invitation: The first step is simply to invite them. A casual conversation can go a long way. Share your enthusiasm about the benefits you've experienced from your exercise routine, whether it's improved energy levels, better mood, or weight loss. Let them know how much more fun it would be to share those experiences with them. You might say, "I've started doing some chair yoga, and I feel so much better! Would you like to join me for a session? It could be a great way for us to catch up!"

Make It Social: Consider organizing a weekly fitness meet-up. This can be as simple as a 30-minute chair yoga session followed by coffee or tea. Making it a social event can be a great way to entice those who may not be as enthusiastic about exercise. Frame it as a time to socialize, relax, and share a few laughs while getting healthier together.

Be Inclusive: Not everyone will be at the same fitness level, and that's perfectly okay. When inviting friends or family, emphasize that the exercises are tailored for everyone, regardless of ability. Chair yoga, for instance, is an excellent option for those who may have mobility issues or are new to fitness. Highlight the adaptability of the exercises, ensuring that everyone feels welcome and included.

Lead by Example: Sometimes, showing is better than telling. Invite them to join you for a session, and demonstrate how enjoyable and accessible the workouts are. Show them modifications for different exercises and reassure them that it's perfectly okay to go at their own pace. Seeing you engage positively with the workout can inspire them to join in.

Use Technology to Your Advantage: In our digital age, many people are more comfortable with virtual connections. Consider inviting friends or family to participate in online classes together. Whether through video calls or fitness apps, you can work out together from the comfort of your own homes. This flexibility can be especially appealing for those who may have transportation issues or prefer to exercise in private.

Plan Special Events: Organize themed fitness events or challenges. For example, you could set up a "30-Day Chair Yoga Challenge" with a prize for participants at the end. This creates excitement and adds a competitive edge to the routine. You can also schedule a monthly outing, like a group walk in the park or a visit to a local wellness fair, which can include gentle exercises and health workshops.

Celebrate Progress Together: As you and your friends or family engage in your fitness journey, take time to celebrate achievements, no matter how small. This could be treating yourselves to a healthy meal together after reaching a fitness goal or simply acknowledging progress with a group chat or call. Celebrating together fosters a sense of community and reinforces the idea that you are all in this journey together.

Offer Encouragement and Support: Sometimes, individuals may hesitate to join due to insecurities or past experiences with exercise. Be sensitive to these feelings and offer encouragement. Share your own challenges and how you overcame them, reassuring them that everyone has their own journey. Remind them that it's about progress, not perfection, and that the goal is to have fun and stay active.

Overcoming Challenges

While encouraging friends and family to join your fitness journey is beneficial, you may encounter some resistance. Some may feel intimidated or think that they don't have time. Address these concerns empathetically:

Addressing Intimidation: Remind them that fitness is a personal journey. Everyone starts somewhere, and there's no need to compare abilities. Emphasize the importance of enjoying the process rather than focusing solely on outcomes.

Time Constraints: Suggest starting with short, manageable sessions that can easily fit into their schedules. Even 15-20 minutes of chair yoga can be beneficial and less daunting.

Physical Limitations: If someone expresses concern about physical limitations, reassure them that chair yoga and modified exercises are designed to accommodate various abilities. Highlight the benefits of moving at their own pace and making adjustments as necessary.

Ultimately, staying connected with friends and family while pursuing fitness can create a supportive, enriching environment. As you encourage others to join your fitness journey, you not only enhance your own experience but also help others improve their health and well-being. This collective effort promotes motivation, accountability, and joy, making the journey of fitness not just about physical transformation but also about fostering relationships that enrich our lives. So, reach out, invite others to join you, and embark on this journey together—because when it comes to fitness, every step is better with a friend.

Conclusion

As we reach the end of this journey through Easy Home Exercises for Seniors Over 60: Chair Yoga with Strength Training to Lose Weight and Gain Flexibility, it's essential to reflect on the path we've traveled together. Adopting a healthier lifestyle is not merely about physical exercise; it's about embracing a holistic approach to well-being that encompasses mind, body, and spirit.

The exercises you've learned—chair yoga and strength training—are not just tools for weight loss or flexibility. They are gateways to renewed vitality and confidence. With each stretch and repetition, you are investing in your health, enhancing your quality of life, and empowering yourself to navigate the challenges that come with aging. Remember, every small step you take contributes to significant changes over time.

Embracing fitness after 60 is not only about maintaining strength and flexibility; it's also about building a supportive community. By involving friends and family in your journey, you create an environment of encouragement, motivation, and shared experiences. Together, you can celebrate milestones, overcome challenges, and enjoy the laughter and joy that come from working out as a team.

As you move forward, carry the knowledge you've gained throughout this book. Incorporate these exercises into your daily routine, listen to your body, and honor its needs. Consistency is key; make fitness a regular part of your life, not just a temporary fix. You may find that, as you progress, your goals evolve. Perhaps you'll discover new interests in movement or explore additional wellness practices like nutrition or mindfulness.

Let this book serve as your guide, a reference point, and a source of inspiration. The journey to health and wellness is lifelong, and it is one that you have the power to shape. Embrace each day as a new opportunity to enhance your strength, improve your flexibility, and nurture your spirit.

Thank you for allowing me to be a part of your fitness journey. I am excited for you as you continue to make strides toward a healthier, more active lifestyle. Remember, it's never too late to start; every moment is a chance to invest in your well-being. Go forward with confidence, resilience, and the knowledge that you have the tools to thrive in your golden years. Here's to a healthier, happier you!

Bonus

Free Workout Videos

INDEX

A

Aging and Exercise, 5, 9, 79
Anti-Inflammatory Smoothies, 151
Arthritis, 29, 108, 118

B

Balance, 13, 17, 23, 26, 79, 108, 174
Bicep Curls, 94, 35
Bone Density, 9, 33, 79

C

Cardiovascular Health, 9, 24, 79
Chair Yoga, 17, 51, 59, 75
Chair-Assisted Squats, 92, 35
Cognitive Function, 11, 25
Core Strength, 35

D

Diet, 135, 138, 141, 144

E

Exercise Myths for Seniors, 26, 27
Exercise Plan, 156, 160, 166, 170, 174
Exercise Readiness, 37

F

Flexibility, 9, 13, 23, 29, 51, 108, 130
Functional Fitness, 17, 33, 35

G

Goal Setting, 43, 40

H

Hip Flexor Stretch, 125
Holistic Fitness Approach, 13, 14

L

Longevity and Well-being, 23
Lower Back Stretch, 121
Low-Carb Meals, 144

M

Mindfulness, 17, 51, 54, 108
Muscle Maintenance, 79, 104

N

Neck Stretch, 115
Nutrition, 135, 141

O

Overhead Press, 98, 35
Osteoporosis, 9, 79, 33

P

Pain Relief, 29, 108, 121
Physical Activity for Seniors, 9, 23, 37
Posture Improvement, 79, 108

R

Recipes for Weight Loss, 144, 148
Resistance Training, 79, 33, 35

S

Sarcopenia, 10, 33
Seated Cat-Cow Stretch, 63
Seated Forward Bend, 65
Seated Hamstring Stretch, 127
Seated Leg Lifts, 89, 35
Seated Mountain Pose, 72
Seated Side Leg Raises, 101
Seated Twist, 68
Strength Training, 13, 79, 33, 104, 35
Stretching for Flexibility, 108, 130

T

Tai Chi, 13, 26
Twists, Seated, 68, 35

W

Weight Loss, 13, 43, 144, 170
Workout Videos (Bonus), 186

www.ingramcontent.com/pod-product-compliance
Lightning Source LLC
Chambersburg PA
CBHW062104220526
45471CB00010B/3590